Lippincott Williams & Wilkins'

Dental Instruments
A Pocket Guide to Identification

Melanie Mitchell, CDA-Emeritus, BGS

Dental Assistant Progam
Wichita Area Technical College
Wichita, Kansas

Total Care Programming, Inc.

SECOND EDITION

Wolters Kluwer | Lippincott Williams & Wilkins
Health

Philadelphia • Baltimore • New York • London
Buenos Aires • Hong Kong • Sydney • Tokyo

Acquisitions Editor: Peter Sabatini
Product Manager: Paula C. Williams
Marketing Manager: Shauna Kelley
Designer: Joan Wendt
Compositor: Aptara, Inc.

Second Edition

Library of Congress Cataloging-in-Publication Data

Mitchell, Melanie, 1953-
  Dental instruments : a pocket guide to identification / Melanie Mitchell, Kathy Booth. – 2nd ed.
    p. ; cm.
  Includes bibliographical references and index.
  ISBN 978-1-60831-638-0 (alk. paper)
  1. Dental instruments and apparatus–Handbooks, manuals, etc.
I. Booth, Kathryn A., 1957- II. Title.
  [DNLM: 1. Dental Instruments–Handbooks. WU 49]
  RK681.M58 2011
  617.60028–dc22
                                        2010037709

DISCLAIMER

CCS1210

This book is dedicated to all of the students who challenge us as educators to continually strive to provide better learning experiences.

A special dedication to my granddaughter Molly (age 2) who keeps me grounded and joyful.

I also wish to thank my husband Larry, my daughter Katie, my son-in-law Jeremy, and my parents Morey and MaryAnn for their patience, ever present support, and encouragement.

About the Author

Melanie Mitchell was employed as a clinical dental assistant in orthodontics and general practice before becoming an instructor and director of the Dental Assistant Program at the Wichita Area Technical College (WATC). Melanie recently retired after 25 years as the director of the Dental Assistant Program and continues to serve as an adjunct instructor at WATC. She has been a DANB Certified Dental Assistant since 1972. She is a life member of the American Dental Assistants Association and has held numerous leadership positions at both the local and state level. Melanie received the American Dental Assistant Association, Sullivan-Schein Award of Excellence in 1999. She has also written, *Clinical Primer: A Pocket Guide for Dental Assistants*, a resource book for use during clinical practice.

Reviewers

- Barbara Adams, CDA, RDH, MA, Program Director, Dental Assisting, Wallace State Community College, Hanceville, AL

- Kimberly G. Bastin, CDA, EFDA, RDH, MS, Dental Assisting Program Director, University of Southern Indiana, Evansville, IN

- Dorothea M. Cavallucci, CDA, EFDA, RDH, MS, Program Director, Dental Assisting/EFDA, Harcum College, Bryn Mawr, PA

- Jane Chandler, RDH, MS, Instructor, Dental Assisting, Tulsa Tech, Tulsa, OK

- Carlos Chavez, BSBM, CDA, RDA, Curriculum Manager, Dental Assistant, Corinthian Colleges, Inc., Santa Ana, CA

- Terri L. Deal, AA, CDA, RDA, Dental Assistant Program Chair, Health and Public Services, Des Moines Area Community College, Ankeny, IA

- Kerri H. Friel, RDH, COA, CDA, BSDH, MA, Assistant Professor, Dental Health Programs, Community College of Rhode Island, Lincoln, RI

- Marie Varley Gillis, RDH, MS, National Dean, Dental Programs, Education Affiliates, Baltimore, MD

- Charmaine Godwin, AA, AS, BA, Med, Assistant Professor, Dental Programs, Santa Fe Community College, Santa Fe, NM

- Gabriele M. Hamm, RDA, CDA, CDPMA, AS, Dental Assisting Instructor/Coordinator, Dental Hygiene/Dental Assisting, Hudson Valley Community College, Troy, NY

- Leora Harty, AAS, CDA, RDA, Instructor, Dental Assistant Program, Medical Careers Institute, Newport News, VA
- Kay W. Hudak, CDA, CDPMA, Instructor, Dental Assisting, Lancaster County Career and Technology Center, Willow Street, PA
- Kay Jukes, RDA, CDA, BS, Instructor and Clinical Coordinator, Dental Assisting, Houston Community College, Houston, TX
- Natalie Kaweckyj, LDA, RF, CDA, CDPMA, COA, COMSA, MADAA, BA, Clinic Coordinator, Children's Dental Services, Minneapolis, MN, President, American Dental Assistants Association, Chicago, IL
- Beth Ladd, CDA, EFDA, Instructor, Dental Assisting, Center for Technology, Essex, Essex Junction, VT
- Janice Lewis, AAHCA, BSHA, EFDA, Program Coordinator and Instructor, Dental Assistant, Pima Medical Institute, Houston, TX
- McMahon, AAS, RDA, CDA, COA, Clinical Instructor, Allied Dental Education, University of Medicine and Dentistry of New Jersey / School of Health Related Professions, Scotch Plains, NJ
- Rhonda Miller, CDA, Dental Program Specialist, Dental Assisting, Pima Medical Institute, Mesa, AZ
- Aamna Nayyar, DDS, Director, Dental Programs, Santa Fe Community College, Santa Fe, NM
- Pamela Nigrelli, CDA, EFDA, Program Director, Dental Assisting, Berks Technical Institute, Wyomissing, PA
- Dawn A. Roberts, Instructor, Allied Health Department, Wor-Wic Community College, Salisbury, MD
- Bobby A. Sconyers, BA, CDA, Dental Assisting Program Coordinator, Dental Education Department, South Florida Community College, Avon Park, FL
- Angela Simmons, BS, Department Chair, Dental Assisting, Fayetteville Technical Community College, Fayetteville, NC

Preface

Identifying dental instruments is essential for every member of the dental team. The small, detailed nature of the instruments and the large number of instruments in dental practice makes learning this skill a daunting task.

This textbook was written in response to needs expressed by dental assisting students. Students asked for a book that was exclusively about dental instruments, that had clear distinctive pictures of the instruments, and that was concisely written. Comprehensive dental textbooks contain descriptions of dental instruments, but they are scattered throughout the textbook and generally are not discussed in as much detail. Students also suggested something that was portable, that they could take home to study or carry with them to the clinical area as a quick reference guide. The result was the first edition of **Dental Instruments: A Pocket Guide to Identification.** With the encouragement of Kathy Booth of Total Care Programming, Inc., a companion CD was developed to provide additional interactive learning experiences. Although this book was written in response to requests of dental assisting students, it is also useful for dental hygiene and beginning dental students.

This second edition includes new chapters of study about instruments used in diagnosis and treatment planning, the dental laboratory, dental radiography, and infection control. The second edition is also enhanced with updated technology, related equipment, tray set-ups for numerous dental procedures, and in-use photos and diagrams.

My book, *Clinical Primer: A Pocket Guide for Dental Assistants,* is another resource book for students as they transition from the classroom to clinical practice. This book and companion CD is a quick reference and review of tooth anatomy, cavity classifications and charting, dental instruments, radiography technique, clinical procedures and tray set-ups, manipulation and usage of dental materials, and Internet resources.

To the Students:

Mastering instrument identification and the organization of instruments and materials for specific procedures is essential for success as a clinical dental auxiliary.

This book is designed to introduce you to instruments by name, function, procedure, and tray set-up. The flash card style can be used in the classroom and for independent study as you master identification of the instruments used in all areas of dentistry. The instrument's image is shown on a separate page facing the description. Once you become familiar with the instruments, the book can be folded over and the images can be used as flashcards for self-testing.

There are 16 *chapters of study* organizing the instruments and equipment by functions and procedures, from basic hand instruments to all specialty areas. The companion CD includes all of the instruments in an interactive format as well as games, crossword puzzles, and other learning activities. Once you are in a clinical setting, the book can continue to be used as a quick reference guide.

Acknowledgments

James Booth, Programming

Kathryn Booth, RN-BSN, RMA (AMT), RPT, CPhT, MS, Instructional Design

Karen M. Callanan, D.D.S., Consultant

Russell L. Coad, D.D.S., Consultant

Thomas J. Foley, D.D.S., Consultant

Cassie McGlynn, Photography

Lourdes Vázquez, CDA, RDH, MS, Consultant

Paula Williams, Product Manager, Lippincott Williams &Wilkins

Patricia Elliot, Permissions

Photo and Illustration Credits

3M Unitek—© 2010 3M. All rights reserved, www.3MUnitek.com
A-dec, www.a-dec.com
AirTechniques, Inc., www.airtechniques.com
American Eagle Instruments®, www.am-eagle.com
Aspetico, www.aseptico.com
Axis® Dental Specialties, www.axisdental.com
Carestream Health Inc., www.kodakdental.com
Coltene Whaledent, www.coltenewhaledent.com
Crosstex, www.crosstex.com
Danville Materials, www.danvillematerials.com
DentalEZ Group, www.dentalez.com
Dentronix, www.dentronix.com
DENTSPLY, www.dentsply.com
DENTSPLY Professional, www.prevent.dentsply.com
DENTSPLY Rinn, www.dentsply.com

DENTSPLY Tulsa Dental Specialties, www.tulsadentalspecialties.com
Dux Dental, www.duxdental.com
GC America, www.gcamerica.com
Gendex Dental Systems, www.gendex.com
Hu-Friedy, www.hf.com
Isolite Systems, www.isolitesystems.com
Lares Research, www.laresdental.com, Karl Schumacher Dental Instruments Company, Inc,
    www.karlschumacher.com
Midmark Corporation, www.midmark.com
Miltex, www.miltex.com
OralCDx®, www.oralcdx.com
Patterson Dental, www.pattersondental.com
Premier Dental Products, www.premusa.com
Professional Results, Inc., www.toothslooth.com
SciCan, www.scican.ca
Shofu Dental Corporation, www.shofu.com
Sirona Dental Systems, www.sirona.com
SybronEndo, www.sybronendo.com
Thermo Scientific, www.thermo.com
Trimira®, www.trimira.com
University of Kentucky College of Dentistry Oral Health Resources

Contents

Chapter 1

Exam and Basic Hand Instruments

INTRODUCTION TO DENTAL HAND INSTRUMENTS

Dental hand instruments are made of metal alloy or plastic resin. They are named according to their use or shape or named for the designer of the instrument.

Hand instruments may be single- or double-ended. Advantages of double-ended: two sizes of the same design in one instrument, two different working ends in one instrument, or two directions of use in one instrument (right/left).

There are three parts of a hand instrument:

1. Working end. The design determines the function and may be a beveled cutting edge (chisel), a point (explorer), a nib (amalgam condenser), a blade (composite instrument) or beaks (pliers).

2. Shank. Portion of the instrument that connects the handle and the working end. The shank may be straight or angled to provide better access to different areas of the mouth.

3. Handle or shaft. Rounded or hexagonal in different diameters and materials for better fit and grip.

1

2

3

MIRROR, MOUTH

FUNCTION: To view tissues of the oral cavity and reflect light for better visibility

FEATURES: Front surface or plane reflective surface. Front surface mirrors reflect from the front of the glass providing a distortion-free reflection.

Mirror sizes #2–#5 (3/4″–15/16″)

Magnifying and double-sided also available

Reusable handles in cone socket or simple stem design

TRAY SET-UP: Exam and Basic Set-up, component of most procedural tray set-ups

CLINICAL APPLICATION: Also used to retract and protect tongue and cheek

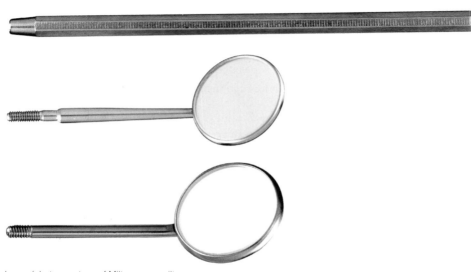

Image/photo courtesy of Miltex, www.miltex.com

5

Basic
1

EXPLORER

FUNCTION: To examine tooth surfaces for caries, calculus, or defects using sense of touch (tactile)

FEATURES: Thin, sharp working end comes in different designs

Common styles are the #1, 2 (pigtail), 11/12, 17, and 23 (Shepard's hook)

May be single- or double-ended (different design on each side)

TRAY SET-UP: Exam and Basic Set-up, component of most procedural tray set-ups

CLINICAL APPLICATION: Also used to:

Check fit of margins of restorations

Evaluate root surfaces and furcation area in periodontal exam (11/12)

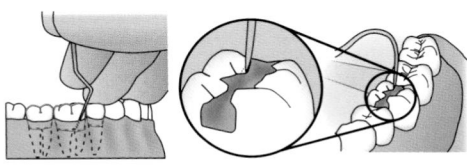

Image modified from University of Kentucky (296m-15, 2-109m)

Remove excess material from restoration or preparation

Remove excess cement

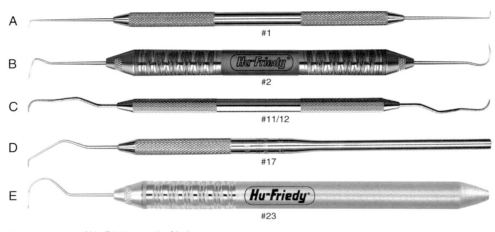

A #1

B #2

C #11/12

D #17

E #23

Images courtesy of Hu-Friedy, www.hu-friedy.com

7

Basic
1

COTTON PLIERS

FUNCTION: To place and remove small objects from the oral cavity (i.e., cotton pellets, root canal instruments, wedges)

FEATURES: Serrated or nonserrated beaks, locking or nonlocking handles

Also known as College pliers or dressing pliers

TRAY SET-UP: Exam and Basic Set-up, component of most procedural tray set-ups

CLINICAL APPLICATION: Also used to retrieve materials from drawers and containers to avoid cross-contamination

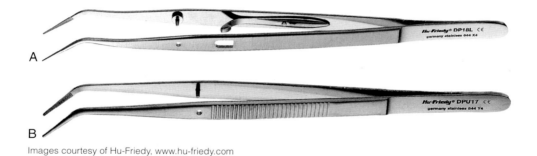

A

B

Images courtesy of Hu-Friedy, www.hu-friedy.com

PERIODONTAL PROBE

FUNCTION: To measure depth of gingival sulcus

FEATURES: Blunt or rounded tip

Flat or cylindrical working end

Line or colored millimeter markings in variety of increments

Metal or plastic in white or yellow with colored markings

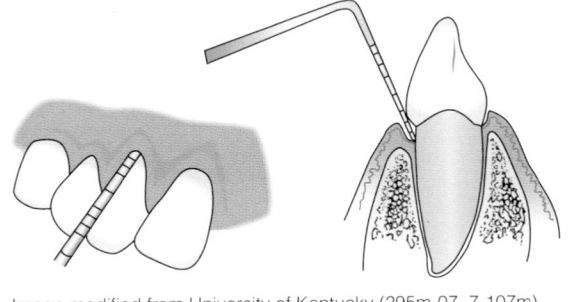

Image modified from University of Kentucky (295m-07, 7-107m)

TRAY SET-UP: Periodontal exam

May be part of Basic Set-up in some offices

CLINICAL APPLICATION: Also used to measure gingival recession

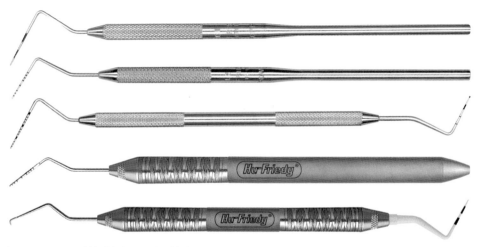

Images courtesy of Hu-Friedy, www.hu-friedy.com

Basic
1

SALIVA EJECTOR TIP

FUNCTION: To remove saliva and maintain dry field using low-volume evacuation

FEATURES: Disposable plastic

Some designed with attached tongue deflector

TRAY SET-UP: Exam and Basic Set-up, component of most procedural tray set-ups. Used primarily when operator is working alone (sealants, coronal polishing, fluoride treatments, taking impressions, cementing crowns)

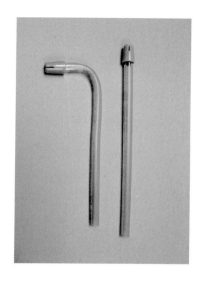

ORAL EVACUATOR TIP

FUNCTION: To maintain a dry working field by removing saliva, blood, and debris with high-volume evacuation

FEATURES: Disposable plastic, sterilizable metal or plastic

Straight or angled with beveled ends

Surgical Aspirator (see Chapter 11 ORAL AND MAXILLOFACIAL SURGERY INSTRUMENTS)

Also known as Aspirator, High Volume Evacuator, Suction, or Vacuum tip

TRAY SET-UP: Exam and Basic Set-up, component of most procedural tray set-ups

CLINICAL APPLICATION: Effective use of oral evacuator reduces microbial aerosols. Also assists in retracting and protecting tongue and cheek. On/off control is located on the suction tubing.

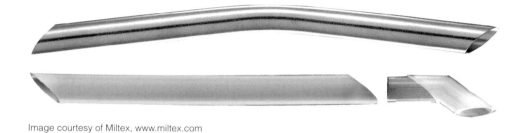

Image courtesy of Miltex, www.miltex.com

Basic
1

ISOLITE, i2 PER MANUFACTURER DRYFIELD

FUNCTION: To provide internal illumination, aspiration, throat protection, and tongue and cheek retraction all in one device

FEATURES: Available in five sizes: pediatric, adult small, adult medium, adult medium deep vestibule, and adult large

Disposable mouthpiece; autoclavable control

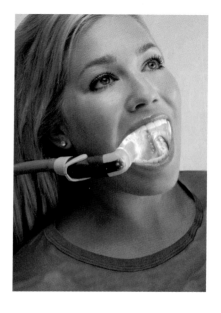

Image courtesy of Isolite Systems, www.isolitesystems.com

ANESTHETIC SYRINGE

FUNCTION: To deliver local anesthesia to intraoral site

FEATURES: Aspirating and Non-aspirating

TRAY SET-UP: Restorative, Fixed Prosthodontic, Endodontic, Periodontic, Oral and Maxillofacial Surgery Treatment Procedures

CLINICAL APPLICATION: An aspirating syringe has a harpoon on the end of the piston, the nonaspirating syringe does not. With pressure, the harpoon imbeds in the rubber stopper of the anesthetic cartridge. As the dentist begins the injection, he/she draws back on the thumb ring, pulling the harpoon and the rubber stopper back and creating a vacuum. This will draw in (aspirate) fluid from the farthest end of the needle. If blood comes back into the cartridge, the dentist will reposition the needle to prevent injecting anesthetic agent into a blood vessel.

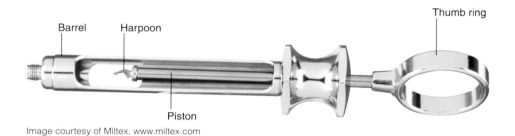

Barrel Harpoon

Thumb ring

Piston

Image courtesy of Miltex, www.miltex.com

Basic
1

19

INTRALIGAMENT SYRINGE

FUNCTION:	Alternative method of delivering local anesthesia; generally to supplement a nerve block. Injection is made in the periodontal ligament space.
FEATURES:	Delivers calibrated amount of anesthetic with each click of the lever
CLINICAL APPLICATION:	Uses 30-gauge short needles and standard 1.8-ml anesthetic cartridges

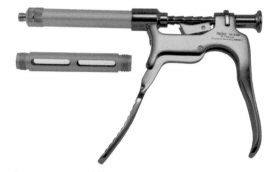

Image courtesy of Miltex, www.miltex.com

Basic
1

LOCAL ANESTHESIA ACCESSORIES

1. Anesthetic needles:

Two lengths—1″ (short) and 1 5/8″ (long)

Three gauges (diameter)—25 gauge, 27 gauge, and 30 gauge

Some manufacturers identify gauge by color-coding caps

Available with plastic or metal hubs

2. Anesthetic cartridges:

Glass vial containing anesthetic solution such as lidocaine (Xylocaine), mepivacaine (Carbocaine), prilocaine (Citanest), and bupivacaine (Marcaine).

Aluminum cap with rubber diaphragm that needle penetrates at one end of cartridge.

Rubber stopper at the other end.

Cartridges are sterile and sealed in "blister packs."

Color coded and labeled with type of anesthetic solution and amount of vasoconstrictor.

3. Recapper: Needles may be used more than one time during a procedure and must be recapped to avoid accidental exposure. For safety, this must be done by using a recapper or the one-handed scoop technique.

4. Sharps container: Needles and other disposable sharps must be disposed of in a labeled, puncture-proof container.

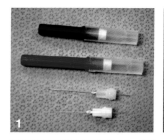

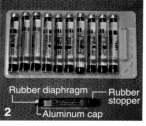

Rubber diaphragm — Rubber stopper
Aluminum cap

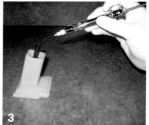

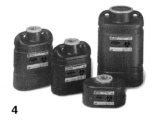

(4) Image courtesy of Crosstex, www.crosstex.com

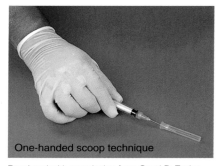

One-handed scoop technique

Reprinted with permission from Carol R. Taylor, Carol Lillis, RN, et al. Fundamentals of Nursing: The Art and Science of Nursing Care. 6th Ed. Philadelphia: Lippincott Williams & Wilkins, 2008.

Basic 1

TRAY SET-UPS

- Assembling all instruments and materials needed for a procedure
- Instruments for a given procedure are sterilized together in a bag or a wrap. Instruments remain in the sterile wrap until the time of use.
- Instruments are arranged on the tray from left to right in their order of use

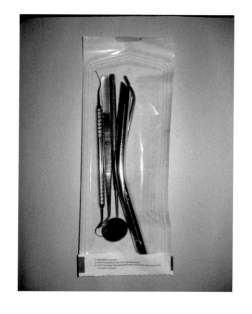

ORAL EXAM AND BASIC SET-UP

1. Mouth mirror
2. Explorer
3. Periodontal probe
4. Cotton pliers
5. Air/water syringe tip
6. Oral evacuator tip
7. Saliva ejector tip
8. 2 × 2 gauze

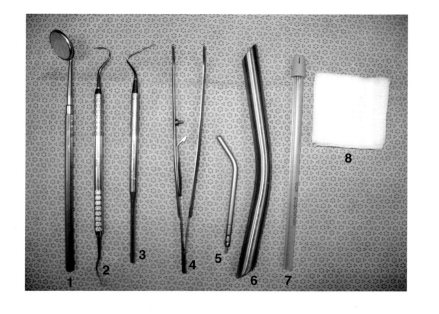

LOCAL ANESTHESIA SET-UP

1. Topical anesthetic
2. Needle recapper
3. 2 × 2 gauze
4. Cotton applicator
5. Anesthetic syringe
6. Anesthetic needle
7. Anesthetic cartridge
8. Air/water syringe tip
9. Oral evacuator tip

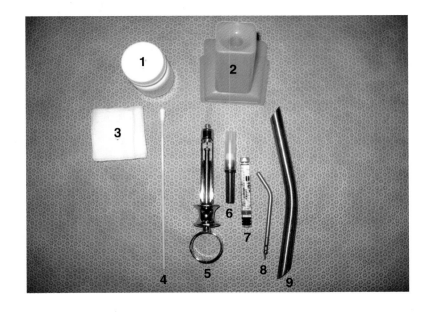

End Chapter 1

CANCER SCREENING SYSTEMS

FUNCTION: To detect abnormal tissue appearance; determine appropriate surgical margins

FEATURES: Handpiece device utilizes three wavelengths, including both reflectance and fluorescence, to visualize abnormal tissue

Trimira® Identafi® 3000 ultra and VELscope light emitting diode (LED) are two of the systems available for oral cancer screening

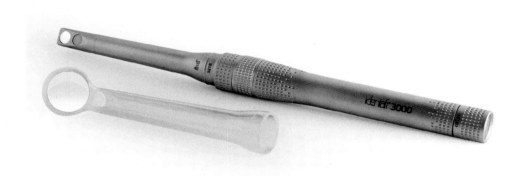

Image courtesy of Trimira®, www.trimira.net

33

OralCDx®

FUNCTION: To obtain a sample of cells from small, white or red intraoral lesions for laboratory analysis

FEATURES: Brush biopsy

Laboratory tissue test

Painless precancer screening (dysplasia) and cancer screening

Minimal or no bleeding

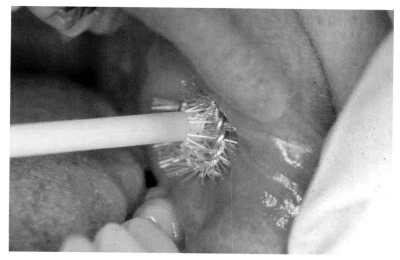

Image courtesy of OralCDx®, www.oralcdx.com

CARIES DETECTION DEVICES

FUNCTION: To aid in early detection of dental caries; indicates decalcification of tooth structure

FEATURES: Handpiece device utilizes light waves (laser, LED, or infrared) and fluorescence to distinguish between healthy tooth tissue and diseased tooth tissue

Kavo DIAGNOdent, Air Techniques Spectra and Midwest Caries I.D.™ are several of the instruments available to aid in caries detection

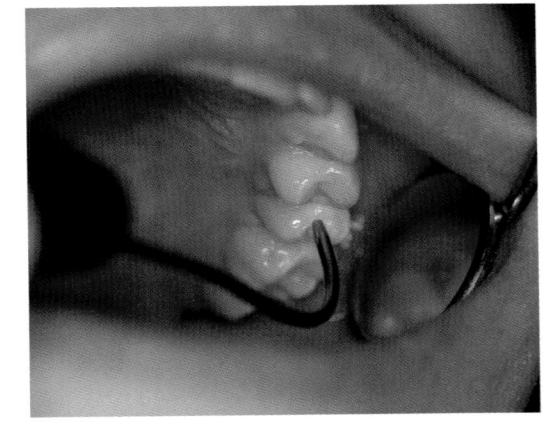

Image courtesy of Dentsply Professional, www.prevent. dentsply.com

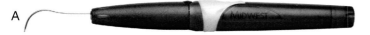

A

Midwest Caries I.D.™ image courtesy of Dentsply Professional,
www.prevent.dentsply.com

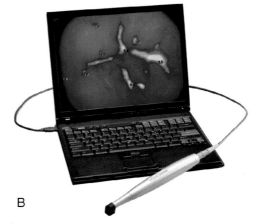

B

Spectra image courtesy of Air Techniques, Inc.,
www.airtechniques.com

LOUPES

FUNCTION: Enhances ability to see small structures and minute detail

Improves accuracy and effectiveness during treatment procedures

FEATURES: Optical device

Provides magnification

Available in clip on loupes (attach to safety glasses or headband) or through-the-lens loupes (optics built into lens of eyeglasses)

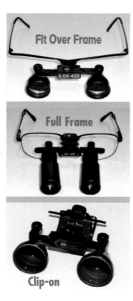

Fit Over Frame

Full Frame

Clip-on

Image courtesy of Vision USA, a Dentrex Company, www.visionusa.biz

Diagnostic & Treatment
2

FIBEROPTIC HEADLIGHT

FUNCTION: Provides direct illumination to the oral cavity enhancing visualization of the treatment area

FEATURES: High intensity LED light source

Battery powered

attaches to loupes or headband

Light intensity control

Filters available to prevent premature curing of composite and bonding materials

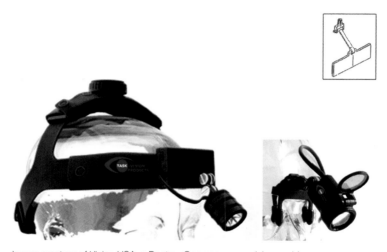

Image courtesy of Vision USA, a Dentrex Company, www.visionusa.biz

TOOTH SLOOTH®

FUNCTION: Diagnostic device to aid in detection of tooth fractures

FEATURES: Sterilizable plastic bite stick

Indentation on domed working end concentrates biting force on one cusp

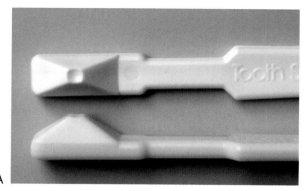

A

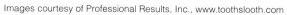
Images courtesy of Professional Results, Inc., www.toothslooth.com

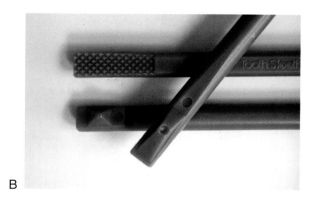

B

INTRAORAL CAMERA

FUNCTION: To illuminate and visualize teeth and oral structures

Used for treatment planning and patient education

FEATURES: LED camera in lightweight handpiece

Images viewed on computer monitor

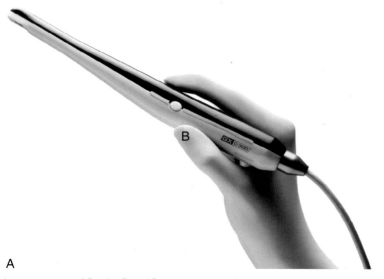

A

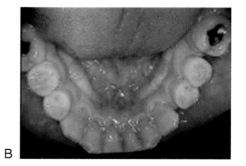

B

Images courtesy of Gendex Dental Systems, www.gendex.com

LIP AND CHEEK RETRACTORS

FUNCTION: To retract lips and cheeks for unobstructed view especially for intraoral photography

TRAY SET-UP: Examination, especially in cosmetic case presentations and orthodontics

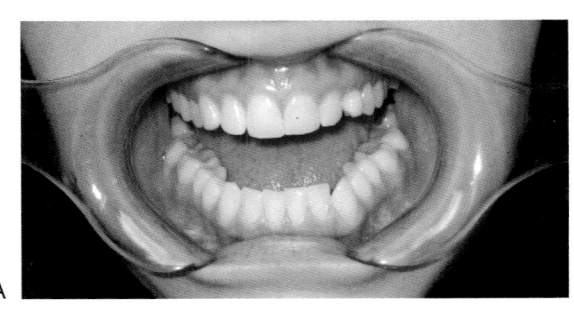

A

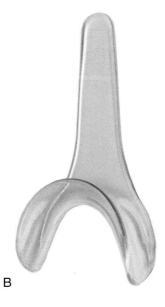

B

Images courtesy of Hu-Friedy, www.hu-friedy.com

End Chapter 2

Chapter 3

Hand Cutting Instruments— Cavity Preparation

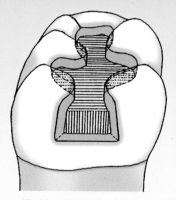

Image modified from University of Kentucky 551m-10

SPOON EXCAVATORS

FUNCTION: To remove soft decay and other materials such as temporary restorations and cement from tooth

FEATURES: Rounded, scoop-like working end

Multiple sizes in "spoon" or "blade" shape

Design of instrument makes it useful for many tasks

TRAY SET-UP: Amalgam, composite, crown and bridge

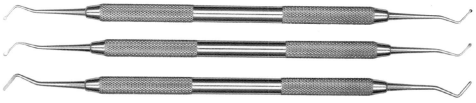

Images courtesy of Hu-Friedy, www.hu-friedy.com

ENAMEL HATCHET

FUNCTION:	To remove decay and refine cavity preparation
FEATURES:	Right and left designs
	Several sizes of width and length of blade
	Usually double ended (right end, left end)
TRAY SET-UP:	Amalgam, composite
CLINICAL APPLICATION:	The use of hand cutting instruments for cavity preparation has declined with improvements in rotary instrument design and changes in restorative techniques. Use is dependent upon individual dentist's preferences.

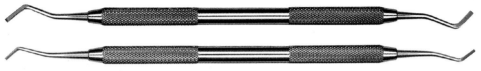

Images courtesy of Hu-Friedy, www.hu-friedy.com

Hand Inst - Cavity Prep 3

STRAIGHT CHISEL

FUNCTION:	To remove decay and refine cavity preparation; pushing motion
FEATURES:	Straight shank Working end in several widths
TRAY SET-UP:	Amalgam, composite
CLINICAL APPLICATION:	The use of hand cutting instruments for cavity preparation has declined with improvements in rotary instrument design and changes in restorative techniques. Use is dependent upon individual dentist's preferences.

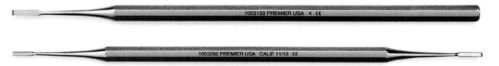

Images courtesy of Premier Dental Products, www.premusa.com

BINANGLE CHISEL

FUNCTION: To remove decay and refine cavity preparation; pushing motion

FEATURES: Angled shank

Working end in several widths

TRAY SET-UP: Amalgam, composite

CLINICAL APPLICATION: The use of hand cutting instruments for cavity preparation has declined with improvements in rotary instrument design and changes in restorative techniques. Use is dependent upon individual dentist's preferences.

Images courtesy of Premier Dental Products, www.premusa.com

WEDELSTAEDT CHISEL

FUNCTION: To remove decay and refine cavity preparation; pushing motion

FEATURES: Curved shank

Working end in several widths

TRAY SET-UP: Amalgam, composite

CLINICAL APPLICATION: The use of hand cutting instruments for cavity preparation has declined with improvements in rotary instrument design and changes in restorative techniques. Use is dependent upon individual dentist's preferences.

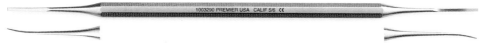

Images courtesy of Premier Dental Products, www.premusa.com

HOE EXCAVATOR

FUNCTION:	To remove decay and refine cavity preparation; pulling motion
FEATURES:	Variety of angled shanks
	Several sizes of width and length of blade
TRAY SET-UP:	Amalgam, composite
CLINICAL APPLICATION:	The use of hand cutting instruments for cavity preparation has declined with improvements in rotary instrument design and changes in restorative techniques. Use is dependent upon individual dentist's preferences.

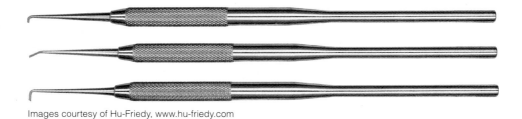

Images courtesy of Hu-Friedy, www.hu-friedy.com

61

ANGLE FORMER

FUNCTION: To remove decay and refine cavity preparation especially line angles and point angles; pushing motion

FEATURES: Angled cutting edge

Angled shank

Several sizes of width and length of blade

TRAY SET-UP: Amalgam, composite

CLINICAL APPLICATION: The use of hand cutting instruments for cavity preparation has declined with improvements in rotary instrument design and changes in restorative techniques. Use is dependent upon individual dentist's preferences.

Images courtesy of Premier Dental Products, www.premusa.com

1003301 PREMIER USA CALIF 32/33 CE

GINGIVAL MARGIN TRIMMER

FUNCTION: To remove decay and refine cavity preparation, especially to bevel the gingival margin of the cavity preparation

FEATURES: Similar to enamel hatchet except that the blade is curved

Mesial and distal margin trimmers

Right and left designs

Several sizes of width and length of blade

Usually double ended (right end, left end)

TRAY SET-UP: Amalgam, composite

CLINICAL APPLICATION: The use of hand cutting instruments for cavity preparation has declined with improvements in rotary instrument design and changes in restorative techniques. Use is dependent upon individual dentist's preferences.

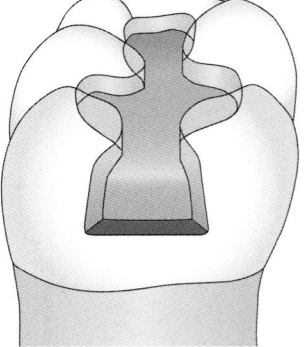

Image modified from University of Kentucky 551m-10

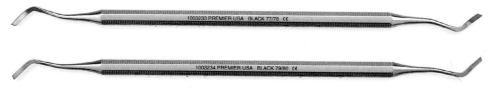

Images courtesy of Premier Dental Products, www.premusa.com

End Chapter 3

Restorative
Instruments

AMALGAM CARRIERS

FUNCTION:	To pick up, carry to, and place amalgam in prepared cavity
FEATURES:	Sizes of working end: mini, regular, large, and jumbo
	Single and double ended
	Lever or syringe style
TRAY SET-UP:	Amalgam
CLINICAL APPLICATION:	After mixing (triturating) alloy and mercury, amalgam is placed in amalgam well or on cotton squeeze cloth for loading the amalgam carrier

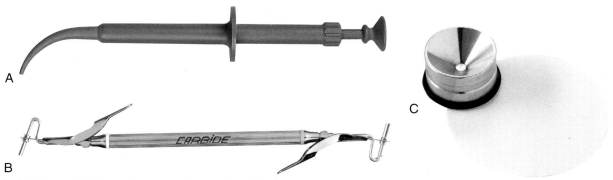

(A) Syringe style amalgam carrier courtesy of Premier Dental Products, www.premusa.com, (B) Lever style amalgam carrier and (C) amalgam well and squeeze cloth courtesy of Patterson Dental, www.pattersondental.com

Restorative
4

Restorative 4

AMALGAM CONDENSERS

FUNCTION: To compact amalgam in the cavity preparation

FEATURES: Working ends are called "nibs"

Various sizes and shapes of working end: round, oval, diamond, rectangular

Smooth or serrated tips

Single and double ended

Also known as amalgam plugger

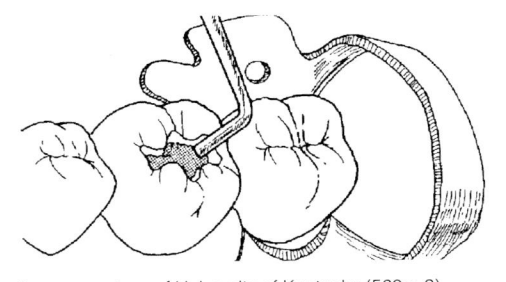

Image courtesy of University of Kentucky (560m-3)

TRAY SET-UP: Amalgam

CLINICAL APPLICATION: Once amalgam hardens on an instrument, it is very difficult to remove. It is important to remove any remaining bits of amalgam from the working ends before cleaning and sterilization.

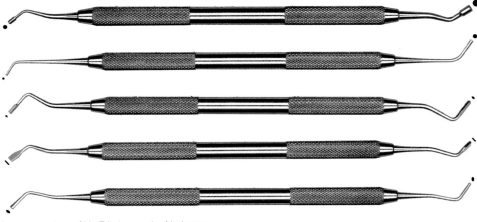

Images courtesy of Hu-Friedy, www.hu-friedy.com

Restorative
4

BURNISHER—BALL

FUNCTION: To smooth and shape metal restorations (amalgams), smooth rough margins (temporary crowns), and shape metal matrix bands

FEATURES: Round ball working end

Often double ended with two sizes

TRAY SET-UP: Amalgam, crown and bridge preparation

Image courtesy of Premier Dental Products, www.premusa.com

73

BURNISHER—POINTED BALL

Also known as "Anatomical Carver" or acorn burnisher

FUNCTION: To smooth and shape metal restorations (amalgams)

FEATURES: Pointed ball working end
Often double ended with two sizes

TRAY SET-UP: Amalgam

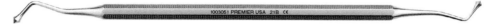

Image courtesy of Premier Dental Products, www.premusa.com

BURNISHER—FOOTBALL

FUNCTION: To smooth and shape metal restorations (amalgams), smooth rough margins (temporary crowns), and shape metal matrix bands

FEATURES: Football-shaped working end

Often double ended with two sizes

TRAY SET-UP: Amalgam, crown and bridge preparation

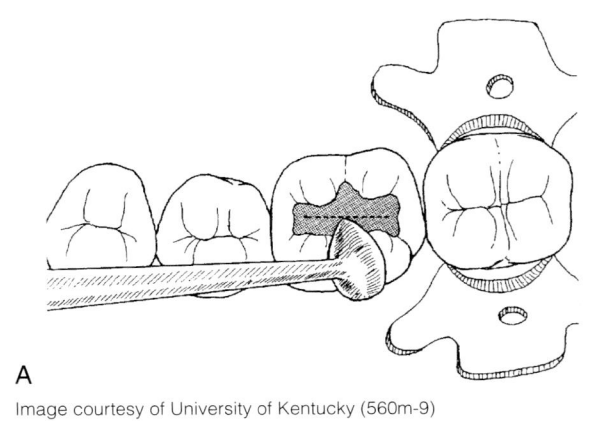

A

Image courtesy of University of Kentucky (560m-9)

B

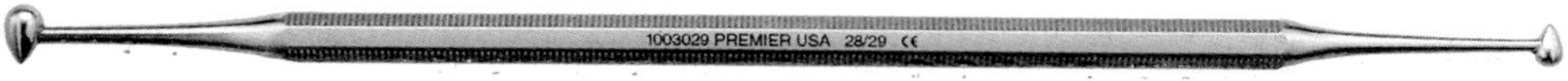

Image courtesy of Premier Dental Products, www.premusa.com

Restorative
4

BURNISHER—T-BALL

FUNCTION:	To smooth and shape metal restorations (amalgams), smooth rough margins (temporary crowns), and shape metal matrix bands
FEATURES:	"T" shaped working end with small ball on one side of "T" and paddle on the other
TRAY SET-UP:	Amalgam, crown and bridge preparation

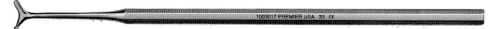

Image courtesy of Premier Dental Products, www.premusa.com

BURNISHER—BEAVERTAIL

FUNCTION: To smooth and shape metal restorations

FEATURES: Paddle like working end
Often double ended with two sizes

TRAY SET-UP: Amalgam

Image courtesy of Premier Dental Products, www.premusa.com

AMALGAM CARVERS—DISCOID-CLEOID

FUNCTION: To remove excess and carve anatomy in amalgam or wax

FEATURES: Discoid—disc-shaped end

Cleoid—pointed, spade-shaped end

TRAY SET-UP: Amalgam

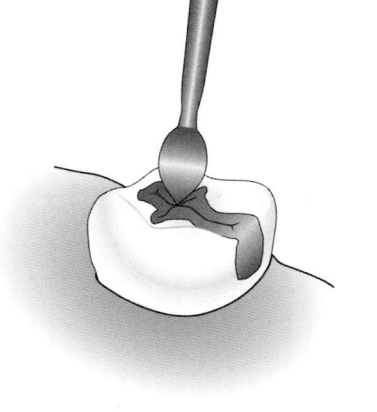

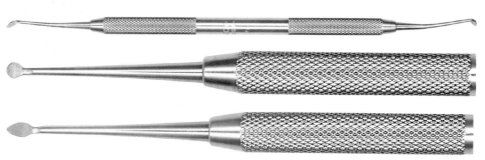

Images courtesy of Hu-Friedy, www.hu-friedy.com

AMALGAM CARVERS—HOLLENBACK CARVER

FUNCTION:	To remove excess and carve anatomy in amalgam or wax
FEATURES:	Paddle-like working ends with thin edges
	Two sizes—smaller version is called a Half Hollenback
TRAY SET-UP:	Amalgam

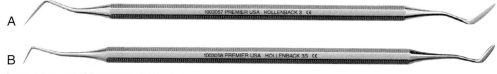

A

B

Images courtesy of Premier Dental Products, www.premusa.com

PLASTIC INSTRUMENT

FUNCTION:	To place moldable ("plastic") restorative materials and cements in the cavity preparation
FEATURES:	Double ended with a non-cutting blade on each end or a nib on one end and a blade on the other
	Many varieties in shape and size
	Made of metal or plastic
TRAY SET-UP:	Amalgam, composite, and temporary restoration

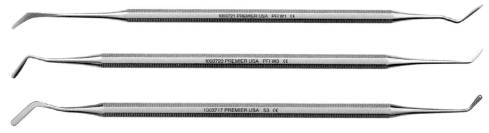

Images courtesy of Premier Dental Products, www.premusa.com

COMPOSITE INSTRUMENT

FUNCTION: To place composite restorative materials in the cavity preparation

Essentially a plastic instrument made of nonstick metal (anodized aluminum or titanium nitride) or made of plastic to prevent sticking, scratching, and discoloration of the composite

FEATURES: Double ended with a non-cutting blade on each end or a nib on one end and a blade on the other

Many varieties in shape and size

TRAY SET-UP: Composite

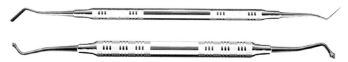

Images courtesy of American Eagle Instruments®, Inc., www.am-eagle.com

Restorative
4

CARVING KNIFE

FUNCTION: To remove excess filling material, "flash"

FEATURES: Thin, sharp blade designed to provide access to interproximal and other tooth surfaces

TRAY SET-UP: Composite

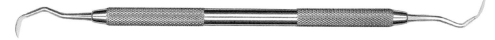

Image courtesy of Hu-Friedy, www.hu-friedy.com

CAVITY LINER APPLICATOR

FUNCTION: To mix and place cavity liner material (calcium hydroxide, glass ionomer) in prepared cavity

FEATURES: Very small ball working end

Single or double ended

TRAY SET-UP: Amalgam, composite

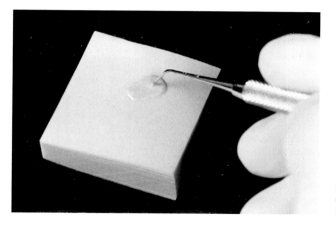

MATRIX BANDS AND RETAINERS—TOFFLEMIRE MATRIX

FUNCTION: A matrix band is used when a mesial or distal tooth surface is missing. It provides a replacement wall to help contour restorative materials during placement.

FEATURES: Metal bands in various gauges and widths

The retainer holds the band tightly around the tooth

Wooden or plastic wedge adapts the band firmly to the proximal tooth surface.

TRAY SET-UP: Amalgam, composite

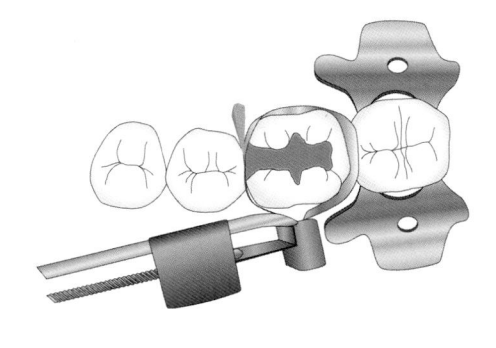

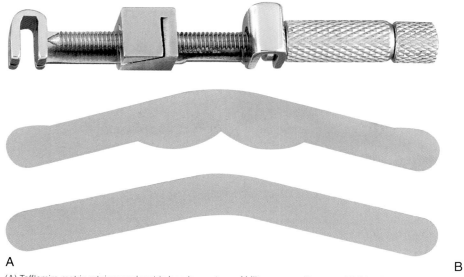

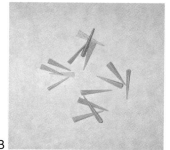

(A) Tofflemire matrix retainer and matrix bands courtesy of Miltex, www.miltex.com (B) Wooden wedges

95

MATRIX BANDS AND RETAINERS—SECTIONAL CONTACT MATRIX

FUNCTION: A matrix band is used when a mesial or distal tooth surface is missing. It provides a replacement wall to help contour restorative materials during placement.

FEATURES: Sectional matrix in several sizes and shapes

An oval ring holds the kidney-shaped matrix in place

Wooden or plastic wedge adapts the band firmly to the proximal tooth surface

TRAY SET-UP: Amalgam, composite

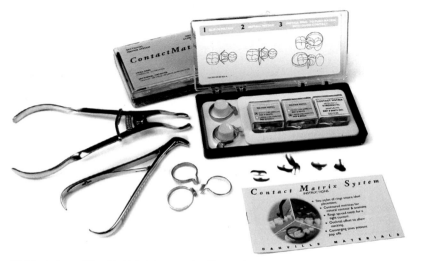

Image courtesy of Danville Materials, www.danvillematerials.com

FUNCTION: A matrix band is used when a mesial or distal tooth surface is missing. It provides a replacement wall to help contour restorative materials during placement.

FEATURES: Preloaded bands

Retainerless system—band tightened with Automate® tightening device

Multiple matrix heights and gauges

Wooden or plastic wedge adapts the band firmly to the proximal tooth surface

TRAY SET-UP: Amalgam

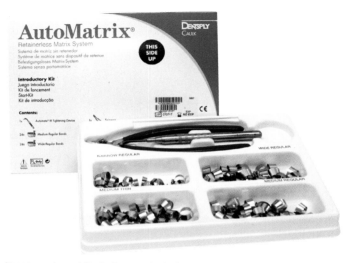

Image courtesy of Dentsply, www.dentsply.com

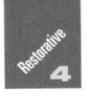

MATRIX BANDS AND RETAINERS—PLASTIC MATRIX STRIP AND HOLDER

FUNCTION: A matrix band is used when a mesial or distal tooth surface is missing. It provides a replacement wall to help contour restorative materials during placement.

FEATURES: Plastic matrix strip used for anterior composite restorations

TRAY SET-UP: Composite

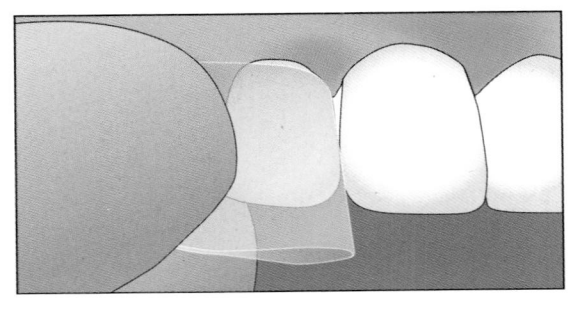

Image modified from University of Kentucky (568m-6)

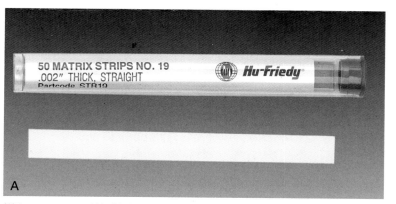

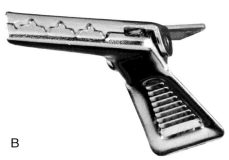

(A) Image courtesy of Hu-Friedy, www.hu-friedy.com, and (B) image courtesy of Miltex, www.miltex.com

ARTICULATING PAPER FORCEPS

FUNCTION: To hold articulating paper over the occlusal surface for checking a patient's occlusal contacts

TRAY SET-UP: Amalgam, composite, crown and bridge

ALSO KNOWN AS: Miller forceps

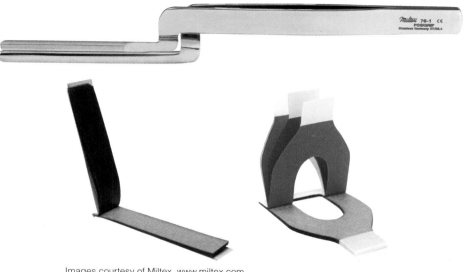

Images courtesy of Miltex, www.miltex.com

103

RESTORATIVE EQUIPMENT

1. AMALGAMATOR:	Mixes amalgam and other restorative materials supplied in premeasured capsules
2. CURING LIGHT:	High intensity light to cure resin materials (composite restoratives, sealants, resin cement) and activate other light-activated materials (bleach)
	LED and halogen technology
	Corded and cordless
3. COMPOSITE DISPENSING GUN:	Device to dispense restorative materials from unidose compules into tooth preparations

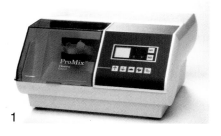

1

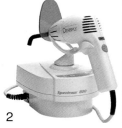

2

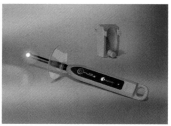

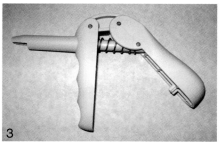

3

Images courtesy of Dentsply, www.dentsply.com

CAVITY PREPARATION AND AMALGAM SET-UP

PURPOSE: To provide instrumentation for removing decay and shaping a cavity to hold a restorative material. This material is contoured to restore normal anatomical form.

1. Basic set-up
2. Local anesthesia set-up
3. Tofflemire matrix band, retainer, and wedges
4. Amalgam well
5. Amalgam capsule
6. Cavity preparation burs
7. Spoon excavator
8. Binangle chisel, enamel hatchet (preference of dentist)
9. Amalgam carrier
10. Amalgam condenser
11. Hollenback carver
12. Discoid/cleoid
13. Ball burnisher
14. Hemostat
15. Articulating paper forceps
16. Handpieces (high and low speed)
17. Cavity base/liner
18. Mixing pad and instrument

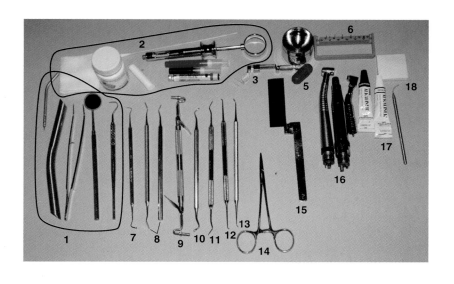

CAVITY PREPARATION AND COMPOSITE SET-UP

PURPOSE: To provide instrumentation for removing decay and shaping a cavity to hold a restorative material. This material is contoured to restore normal anatomical form.

1. Basic set-up
2. Local anesthesia set-up
3. Cavity preparation burs
4. Spoon excavator
5. Binangle chisel, enamel hatchet (preference of dentist)
6. Composite placement instrument
7. Applicator for bonding agent
8. Acid etch
9. Plastic matrix band
10. Bonding agent and disposable well
11. Articulating paper forceps
12. Abrasive strip
13. Abrasive discs and polishing points
14. Handpieces (high and slow speed)
15. Composite compule and dispensing gun

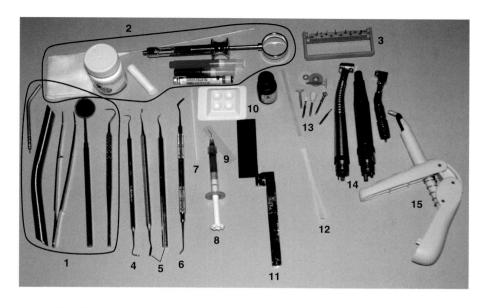

Restorative
4

End Chapter 4

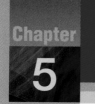

Dental Dam
Instruments

INDICATIONS FOR THE DENTAL DAM

A **dental dam** is placed during restorative and endodontic procedures to:

Provide moisture control

Retract gingiva, cheek, and tongue for increased visibility and accessibility of the treatment area

Protect the patient from contact with irritating materials

Prevent the patient from swallowing debris

Reduce the dental team's contact with oral microbes

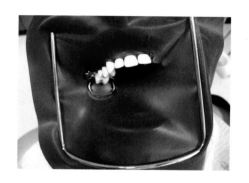

Dental Dam
5

DENTAL DAM MATERIAL

FUNCTION: Flexible barrier to isolate the operating field

VARIETIES: Latex and nonlatex

5 × 5 or 6 × 6

Thin, medium, heavy, X-heavy

Light, dark, green, blue, and assorted pastel colors

Also available with built-in frame

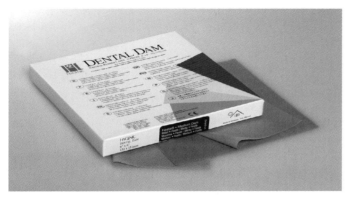

Images courtesy of Coltene Whaledent, www.coltene.com

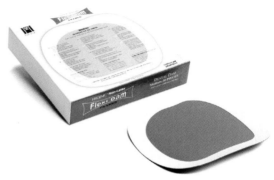

DENTAL DAM TEMPLATE

FUNCTION: To mark tooth position on the dental dam for punch holes

VARIETIES: Circular marks on template correspond to the position and spacing of the teeth in the dental arch

Plastic template or marking stamp

Sized for 5″ or 6″ dam

CLINICAL APPLICATION: Templates are for ideally positioned teeth, and often hole positions must be modified for the individual patient. Templates are helpful when learning but with experience a template may not be necessary.

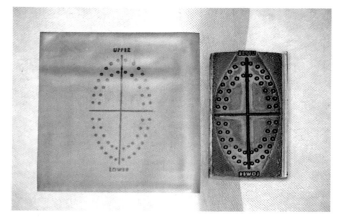

6 X 6 in (15.2 X 15.2 cm)

Image courtesy of Hu-Friedy, www.hu-friedy.com

Reprinted with permission from Gladwin MA, Bagby M. Clinical aspects of dental materials: theory, practice, and cases. 3rd ed. Baltimore, MD: Lippincott Williams & Wilkins, 2008.

Dental Dam
5

DENTAL DAM PUNCH

FUNCTION: To create proper sized holes in the dam to expose the teeth to be isolated

FEATURES: Five punch sizes on a rotating wheel to create holes that are sized correctly for all teeth to be isolated:

No. 5 (largest size punch hole) used for the anchor tooth

No. 4 used for molars

No. 3 used for premolars and canines

No. 2 used for maxillary incisors

No. 1 used for mandibular incisors

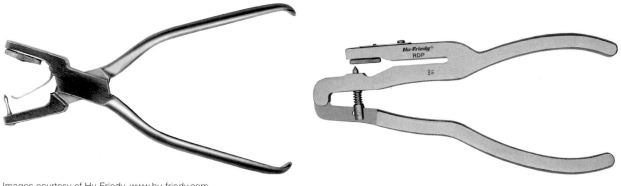

Images courtesy of Hu-Friedy, www.hu-friedy.com

Dental Dam
5

DENTAL DAM CLAMP—WINGED

FUNCTION: To stabilize and hold the dam in place. The clamp is placed on the most distal tooth isolated.

FEATURES: Various sizes and jaw designs to adapt to cervical areas of specific teeth

Extensions, "wings," on the outside of each jaw allow for simultaneous application of the clamp and dam material

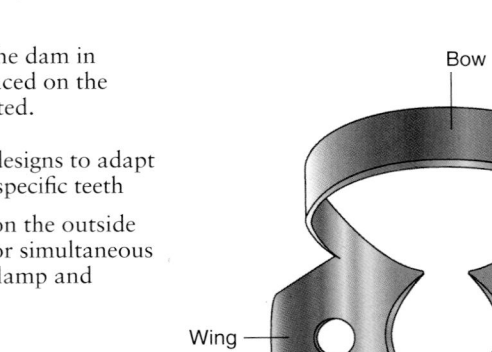

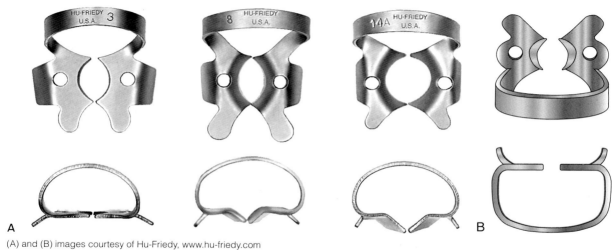

(A) and (B) images courtesy of Hu-Friedy, www.hu-friedy.com

121

Dental Dam
5

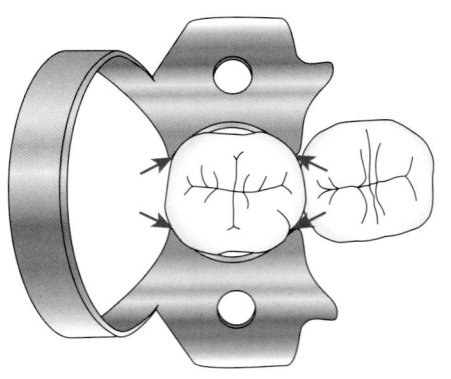

Dental Dam
5

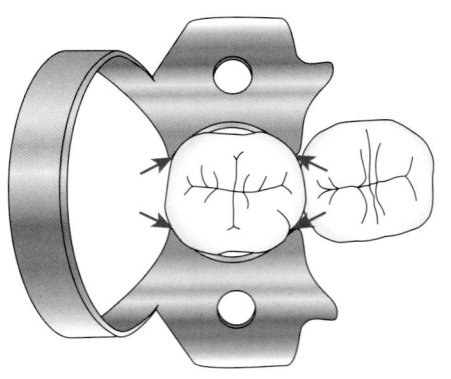

DENTAL DAM CLAMP—WINGLESS

FUNCTION: To stabilize and hold the dam in place. The clamp is placed on the most distal tooth isolated.

FEATURES: Various sizes and designs to adapt to cervical areas of specific teeth

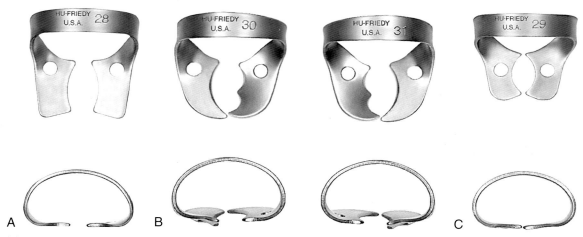

(A) Mandibular molar dental dam clamp, (B) maxillary molar left and right dental dam clamps, and (C) premolar dental dam clamp courtesy of Hu-Friedy, www.hu-friedy.com

Dental Dam
5

DENTAL DAM CLAMP—LABIAL

FUNCTION: To stabilize and hold the dam in place. Labial clamps are used for labial caries on anterior teeth.

FEATURES: Bows on mesial and distal

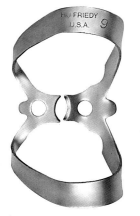
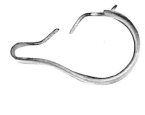

Image courtesy of Hu-Friedy, www.hu-friedy.com

DENTAL DAM CLAMP FORCEPS

FUNCTION: To place and remove the dental dam clamp

FEATURES: Beaks fit into the holes on each jaw of the clamp and spread the clamp slightly to fit over the anchor tooth.

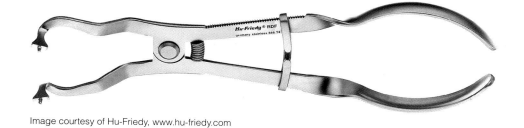

Image courtesy of Hu-Friedy, www.hu-friedy.com

Dental Dam
5

DENTAL DAM FRAME

FUNCTION: Stretches and holds the dam away from the working area outside the mouth

VARIETIES: U-shaped or round

Metal or plastic (radiolucent)

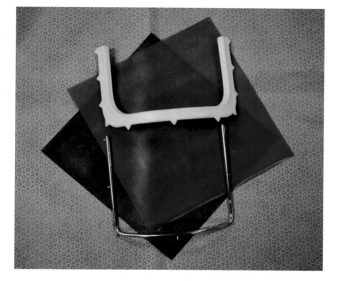

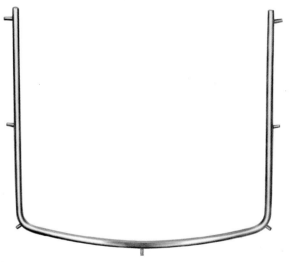

Dental Dam

5

DENTAL DAM SET-UP

PURPOSE: To provide instrumentation for placing a barrier device for moisture control, patient protection, retraction, and reduction of microbes.

1. Dental dam template
2. Dental dam
3. Dental dam frame
4. Dental dam clamps
5. Floss
6. Applicator for lubricant
7. Dental dam punch
8. Dental dam clamp forceps
9. Iris scissors
10. Beavertail burnisher

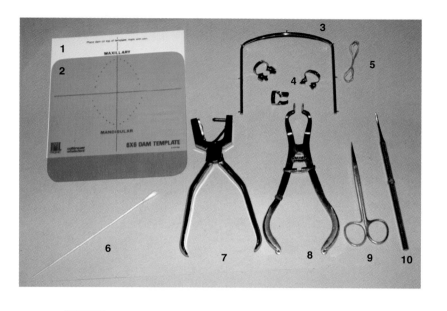

Dental Dam

5

End Chapter 5

Dental
Handpieces

FUNCTION: To hold and rotate cutting instruments (bur, diamond) for removal of decay and tooth structure to form cavity preparations and crown preparations

Accepts burs and other rotary instruments with friction grip (FG) shank

FEATURES: Powered by compressed air supplied through dental unit hoses.

Burs and diamonds are held in place and removed by opening and closing the chuck in the head of the handpiece. This is accomplished by using a bur wrench, a built-in power lever, or a built-in push button chuck.

Fiber optic variation has a light incorporated into the handpiece to illuminate the working area when the handpiece is activated.

TRAY SET-UP: Cavity preparation, crown preparation, and all procedures requiring tooth structure or bone removal

CLINICAL APPLICATION: Dental unit hoses also supply water to handpiece. Water exits the handpiece through an opening just below bur chuck. This protects tooth from damage by heat generated during the cutting process. A switch on the dental unit controls the amount of water output. Speed of handpiece is controlled with a rheostat (foot pedal).

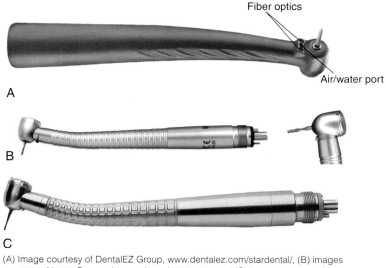

Fiber optics

Air/water port

A

B

C

(A) Image courtesy of DentalEZ Group, www.dentalez.com/stardental/, (B) images courtesy of Lares Research, www.laresdental.com, and (C) image courtesy of Dentsply Professional, www.prevent.dentsply.com

SLOW SPEED HANDPIECE, STRAIGHT

FUNCTION: Used outside the mouth and in the lab to hold rotary instrument for adjusting and smoothing prostheses

With contra-angle attachment, used intraorally to remove decay and tooth tissue to refine cavity preparations, to make adjustments to prostheses, and to adjust and polish restorations

With right-angle attachment, used intraorally to polish teeth and restorations

FEATURES: Accepts rotary instruments with a straight shank as well as contra-angle and right-angle handpiece attachments

TRAY SET-UP: Prophylaxis, crown seat, denture insert, denture adjustment, and cavity preparation refinement

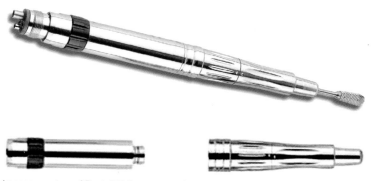

Images courtesy of DentalEZ Group, www.dentalez.com/stardental/

SLOW SPEED HANDPIECE, PROPHY

FUNCTION: To polish teeth (remove soft debris) and polish restorations (smooth and shine) with prophy cups and brushes

FEATURES: Slow speed handpiece

Lighter weight than conventional straight handpiece

Designs: One piece motor and right angle extension—accepts screw-on prophy cups and brushes

DESIGN: Short straight handpiece—accepts right-angle attachment

TRAY SET-UP: Prophylaxis

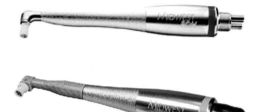

Images courtesy of Dentsply Professional, www.prevent.dentsply.com

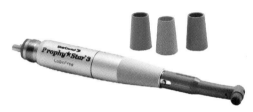

Images courtesy of DentalEZ Group, www.dentalez.com/stardental/

HANDPIECE ATTACHMENT—CONTRA-ANGLE

FUNCTION: Used with straight handpiece to provide better intraoral accessibility

FEATURES: Accepts rotary instruments with latch type shank
Attaches to straight slow-speed handpiece

TRAY SET-UP: Crown seat, denture insert and adjustment, cavity preparation refinement

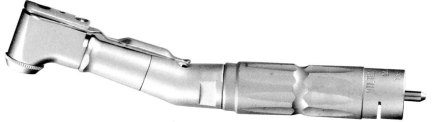

Image courtesy of Miltex, www.miltex.com

HANDPIECE ATTACHMENT—RIGHT ANGLE (PROPHY ANGLE)

FUNCTION: Holds prophy cup or brush to polish teeth and restorations

FEATURES: Attaches to straight slow-speed handpiece
Accepts screw-type rubber cups and brushes
Sterilizable stainless steel or disposable plastic

TRAY SET-UP: Prophylaxis

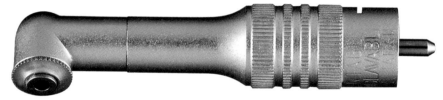

Image courtesy of Miltex, www.miltex.com

ELECTRIC HANDPIECE

FUNCTION: Alternative to compressed air-driven handpieces for cavity preparations and crown preparations; for adjusting dentures, temporary restorations, orthodontic appliances, and splints; and for endodontic procedures

FEATURES: Electric motor with high-speed contra-angle handpiece, straight handpiece, low-speed handpiece, and endodontic handpiece

Increased torque for faster cutting at low speeds

Less noise and vibration than air-driven handpieces

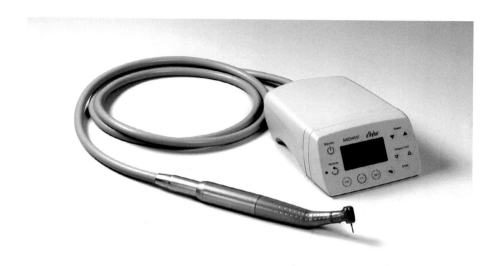

Image courtesy of Dentsply Professional, www.prevent.dentsply.com

AIR ABRASION SYSTEM

FUNCTION: To remove small areas of decayed tooth structure for composite restorations; to prepare tooth surface for sealants; and to etch all metals, composites, and amalgam for bonding

FEATURES: Particles of silica and aluminum oxide are propelled through a handpiece by compressed air to abrade the tooth structure

Less noise and vibration then with conventional high-speed handpiece but can only be used for minimal amount of decay

CLINICAL APPLICATION: Use dental dam to protect surrounding teeth and soft tissue. Use high-volume evacuation throughout procedure to reduce airborne particles

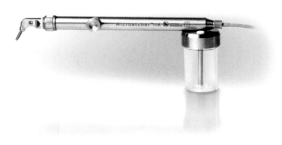

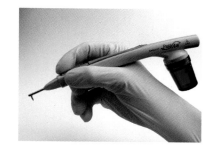

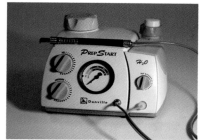

Images courtesy of Danville Materials, www.danvillematerials.com

AUTOMATED HANDPIECE MAINTENANCE DEVICES

FUNCTION: To automatically clean handpiece air/water lines, lubricate air turbines and gears, and expel excess fluid and debris in preparing handpieces for sterilization. Proper cleaning and lubrication reduces performance problems and extends the life of the handpiece.

MODELS AVAILABLE: A-dec Assistina, KaVo QUATTROcare

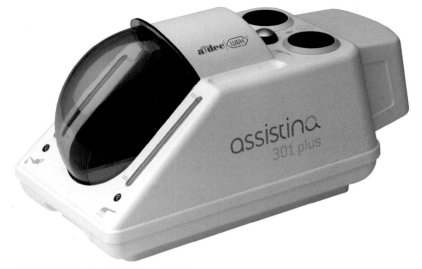

Image courtesy of A-dec, www.a-dec.com

Handpieces
6

HIGH-SPEED HANDPIECE CLEANING AND STERILIZATION—MANUAL OPERATION

While wearing appropriate personal protective equipment after each patient:
Run handpiece, with bur in place, into suction for 20–30 seconds to flush bioburden from interior of handpiece and waterlines.

- Disconnect handpiece from tubing

- In sterilization area, scrub external surface of handpiece with soap and water; dry

- Place paper towel over head of instrument and spray pressurized cleaner/lubricant into the central tube in the back end of the handpiece until ejected solution comes out clean

- Reattach handpiece to air/water system and flush out excess cleaner/lubricant

- Wipe off any excess from handpiece and place in sterilization bag

- Sterilize with steam heat sterilizer

- After sterilization cycle, when cool, open bag just enough to lubricate if recommended by manufacturer

Note: Recommended cleaning and sterilization procedures vary by manufacturer and by model of handpiece. Always read and follow carefully the manufacturer's specific instructions for cleaning, lubrication, and sterilization of handpieces.

Handpieces
6

End Chapter 6

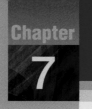

Dental Burs and Rotary Instruments

ROTARY INSTRUMENTS—DENTAL BURS

FUNCTION: Excavation of caries and removal of enamel and dentin to design cavity for a restoration; to smooth and trim restorations; to adjust prosthetic and orthodontic appliances; and to remove and section teeth

FEATURES: Cutting instruments designed to fit into the chuck of a dental handpiece

Burs come in a variety of shapes and sizes and are classified according to use:

- Cavity preparation burs
- Finishing burs
- Laboratory burs
- Surgical burs

PARTS OF A BUR: **1.** Head—the working end (the various head shapes are introduced on the following pages in this section)

2. Neck—the tapered portion that connects the head to the shank

3. Shank—the portion designed to fit into the handpiece

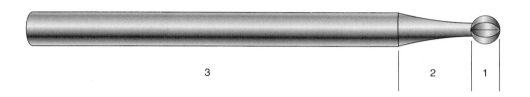

3   2   1

ROTARY INSTRUMENTS—SHANK TYPES

FUNCTION: To insert and hold bur in dental handpiece

Different shank designs are required for different handpieces

SHANK TYPES: 1. Straight or handpiece shank (HP)—used in straight, low speed handpiece

2. Latch type shank (RA/CA/LA)—used in contra-angle handpiece attachment

3. Friction grip shank (FG)—used in high speed, contra-angle handpiece

4. Short friction grip shank (SS)—used in high speed, contra-angle handpiece

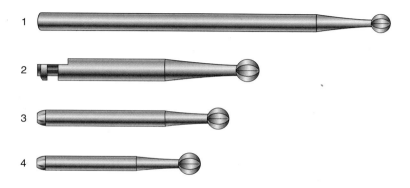

1

2

3

4

157

CAVITY PREPARATION BURS—ROUND

FUNCTION: Excavation of caries; removal of enamel and dentin to design cavity for a restoration; gain access to root canal

FEATURES: Tungsten carbide, 6–8 cutting blades

Sizes: ¼, ½, 1, 2, 3, 4, 5, 6, 7, 8, 10

FG, RA, HP, FG–SS shanks

TRAY SET-UP: Cavity preparation

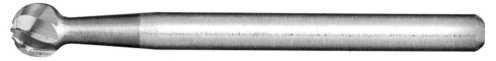

Image courtesy of Miltex, www.miltex.com

159

CAVITY PREPARATION BURS—STRAIGHT FISSURE PLAIN

FUNCTION: Excavation of caries; removal of enamel and dentin to design cavity for a restoration

FEATURES: Tungsten carbide, 6–8 cutting blades

Sizes: 56, 57, 58, 59, 60

FG, RA, HP, FG–SS shanks

TRAY SET-UP: Cavity preparation

Image courtesy of Miltex, www.miltex.com

CAVITY PREPARATION BURS—STRAIGHT FISSURE CROSSCUT

FUNCTION: Excavation of caries; removal of enamel and dentin to design cavity for a restoration

FEATURES: Tungsten carbide, 6–8 cutting blades

Sizes: 556, 557, 558, 559, 560

FG, RA, HP, FG–SS shanks

TRAY SET-UP: Cavity preparation

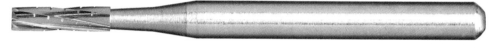

Image courtesy of Miltex, www.miltex.com

163

CAVITY PREPARATION BURS—TAPERED FISSURE PLAIN

FUNCTION: Excavation of caries; removal of enamel and dentin to design cavity for a restoration

FEATURES: Tungsten carbide, 6–8 cutting blades

Sizes: 169, 170, 171, 172

FG, RA, HP, FG–SS shanks

TRAY SET-UP: Cavity preparation

Image courtesy of Miltex, www.miltex.com

CAVITY PREPARATION BURS—TAPERED FISSURE CROSSCUT

FUNCTION: Excavation of caries; removal of enamel and dentin to design cavity for a restoration

FEATURES: Tungsten carbide, 6–8 cutting blades

Sizes: 699, 700, 701, 702, 703

FG, RA, HP, FG–SS shanks

TRAY SET-UP: Cavity preparation

Image courtesy of Miltex, www.miltex.com

167

CAVITY PREPARATION BURS—ROUND END FISSURE

FUNCTION: Excavation of caries; removal of enamel and dentin to design cavity for a restoration

FEATURES: Tungsten carbide, 6–8 cutting blades

Sizes: tapered plain 1169–1172; tapered crosscut 1700–1702; straight plain 1156–1158, straight crosscut 1556–1558

FG, RA, HP, FG–SS shanks

TRAY SET-UP: Cavity preparation

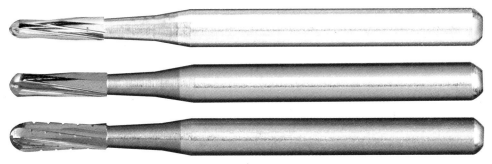

Images courtesy of Miltex, www.miltex.com

CAVITY PREPARATION BURS—INVERTED CONE

FUNCTION: Excavation of caries; removal of enamel and dentin to design cavity for a restoration

FEATURES: Tungsten carbide, 6–8 cutting blades

Sizes: 33½, 34, 35, 36, 37, 38, 39

FG, RA, HP, FG–SS shanks

TRAY SET-UP: Cavity preparation

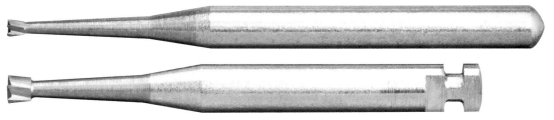

Images courtesy of Miltex, www.miltex.com

171

CAVITY PREPARATION BURS—PEAR

FUNCTION: Excavation of caries; removal of enamel and dentin to design cavity for a restoration

FEATURES: Tungsten carbide, 6–8 cutting blades

Sizes: 329, 330, 331, 332

FG, RA, HP, FG–SS shanks

TRAY SET-UP: Cavity preparation

Image courtesy of Miltex, www.miltex.com

173

CAVITY PREPARATION BURS—WHEEL

FUNCTION: Excavation of caries; removal of enamel and dentin to design cavity for a restoration

FEATURES: Tungsten carbide, 6–8 cutting blades

Sizes: 14

FG, RA, HP, FG–SS shanks

TRAY SET-UP: Cavity preparation

Image courtesy of Miltex, www.miltex.com

175

CAVITY PREPARATION BURS—END CUTTING

FUNCTION:	Excavation of caries; removal of enamel and dentin to design cavity for a restoration
FEATURES:	Tungsten carbide, 6–8 cutting blades
	Sizes: 956, 957
	FG, RA, HP, FG–SS shanks
TRAY SET-UP:	Cavity preparation

Image courtesy of Miltex, www.miltex.com

177

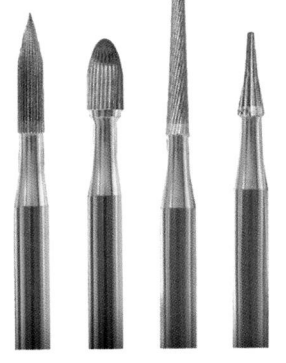

FINISHING BURS

FUNCTION: Contouring, smoothing, and polishing of restorative material

FEATURES: Tungsten carbide, 12 cutting blades

Various shapes and sizes (cone, oval, flame, egg, taper, pear), with more blades (fissures) for smoothing

Mostly FG shank, some are available in RA shank

TRAY SET-UP: Cavity preparation

Image courtesy of Dentsply Professional, www.prevent.dentsply.com

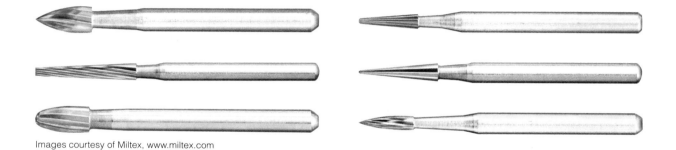

Images courtesy of Miltex, www.miltex.com

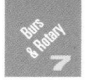

LABORATORY BURS

FUNCTION: To adjust, trim, and smooth prosthetic and orthodontic appliances

FEATURES: Various shapes and sizes (round, flame, barrel, pear) with straight shanks and large working ends

TRAY SET-UP: Denture and appliance adjustment

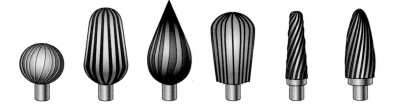

181

**Burs
& Rotary**
7

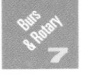

SURGICAL BURS

FUNCTION:	To remove bone and section teeth
FEATURES:	Various shapes and sizes with extra long, straight shanks
TRAY SET-UP:	Impaction, tooth extraction

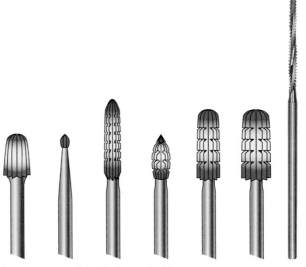

Image courtesy of Hu-Friedy, www.hu-friedy.com

183

DIAMONDS

FUNCTION: For rapid, bulk reduction of tooth structure, polishing and finishing restorations (fine), bone and gingival contouring in periodontal surgical procedures (coarse)

FEATURES: Various shapes and sizes (cone, oval, flame, egg, taper, pear, wheel, discs, strip)

TRAY SET-UP: Crown and bridge preparation, cavity preparation, gingivoplasty, alveoplasty

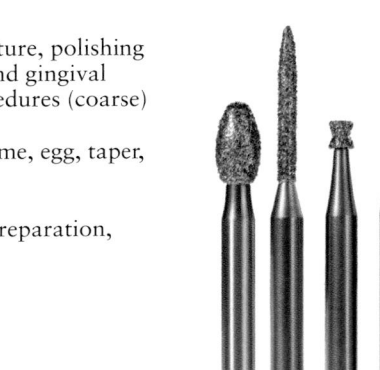

Image courtesy of Dentsply Professional, www.prevent.dentsply.com

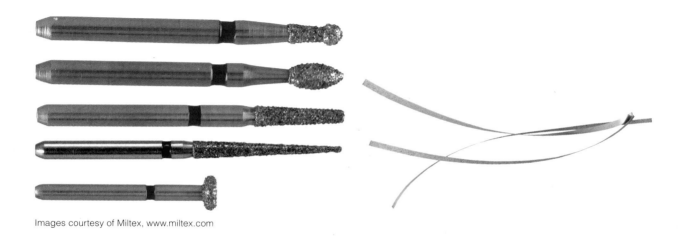

Images courtesy of Miltex, www.miltex.com

185

MANDREL—SCREW ON

FUNCTION: To mount discs, wheels, stones for use in a handpiece
Used in the laboratory and at chairside

FEATURES: Mount for discs and wheels with pinhole centers
Mostly HP and RA shanks, some available in FG shank

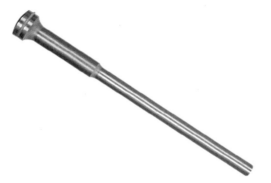

Image courtesy of Shofu Dental Corporation, www.shofu.com

MANDREL—SNAP ON

FUNCTION: To mount discs for use in a handpiece

FEATURES: Mount for discs with brass centers
Mostly HP and RA shanks, some available in FG shank

TRAY SET-UP: Composite restoration

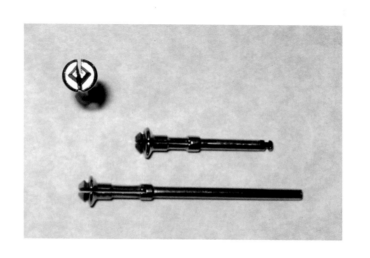

SANDPAPER ABRASIVES

FUNCTION: To shape and smooth restorations

FEATURES: Discs (snap on and screw on) and strips

Various sizes, grits, and abrasive materials
(aluminum oxide, garnet, sand, cuttle)

TRAY SET-UP: Composite restoration

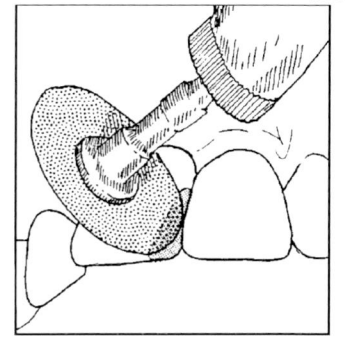

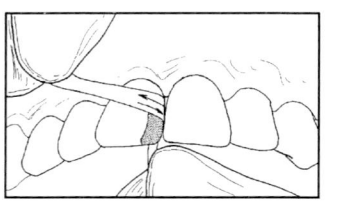

Image courtesy of University of Kentucky (569m-17, 569m-20)

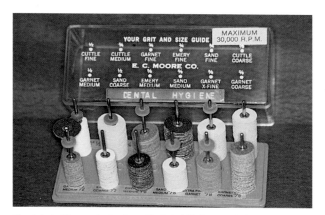
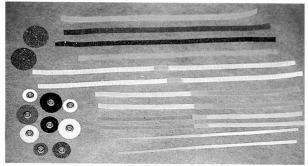

Reprinted with permission from Gladwin MA, Bagby M. Clinical aspects of dental materials: theory, practice, and cases. 3rd ed. Baltimore, MD: Lippincott Williams & Wilkins, 2008.

COMPOSITE FINISHING SYSTEM

FUNCTION: To shape, smooth, and polish composite restorations

FEATURES: Flexible discs designed specifically for composite

Disc covers top of mandrel to prevent damage to restoration

Color-coding designates grit

Multiple manufacturers

TRAY SET-UP: Composite restoration

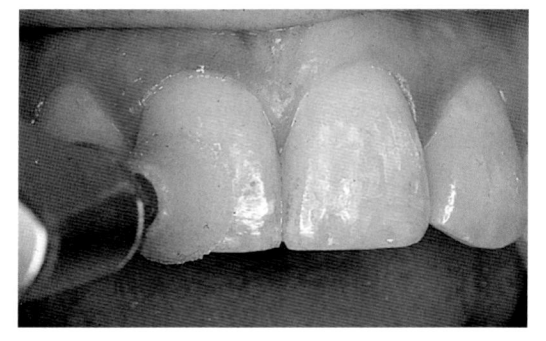

Reprinted with permission from Gladwin MA, Bagby M. Clinical aspects of dental materials: theory, practice, and cases. 3rd ed. Baltimore, MD: Lippincott Williams & Wilkins, 2008.

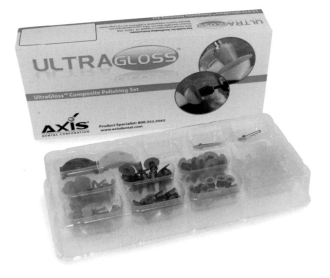

Image courtesy of Axis® Dental Specialties, www.axisdental.com

STONES

FUNCTION: Made of silicon carbide or aluminum oxide to smooth, trim, and polish amalgam, gold, composite, acrylic, porcelain

Used in the laboratory and at chairside

FEATURES: Various shapes, sizes, grits

Green, red, pink, blue, yellow, white, gray, brown points/stones

Mounted on shanks or unmounted to attach to mandrel

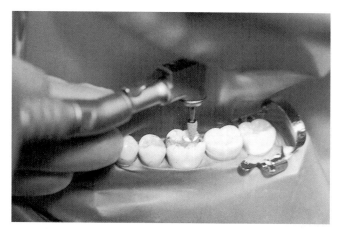

Reprinted with permission from Gladwin MA, Bagby M. Clinical aspects of dental materials: theory, practice, and cases. 3rd ed. Baltimore, MD: Lippincott Williams & Wilkins, 2008.

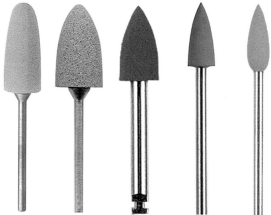

Image courtesy of Axis® Dental Specialties, www.axisdental.com

RUBBER ABRASIVES—WHEEL AND DISK

FUNCTION:	To finish and polish ceramics, composites, alloy, and gold intraorally and in the lab
FEATURES:	Various sizes and grits
	Mounted and unmounted
	Green, red, pink, blue, yellow, white, gray, brown
TRAY SET-UP:	Restorative, crown and bridge

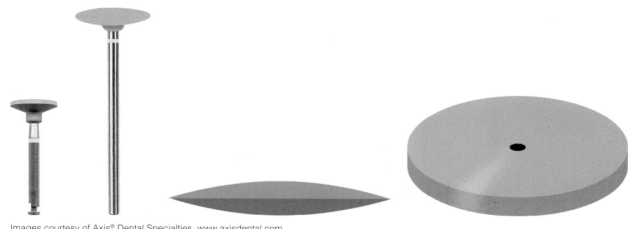

Images courtesy of Axis® Dental Specialties, www.axisdental.com

Burs
& Rotary

RUBBER ABRASIVES—POINT AND CUP

FUNCTION: To finish and polish ceramics, composites, alloy, and gold intraorally and in the lab

FEATURES: Various sizes, shapes and grits

Mounted to HP, RA, and FG shanks

Green, red, pink, blue, yellow, white, gray, brown

TRAY SET-UP: Restorative, crown and bridge

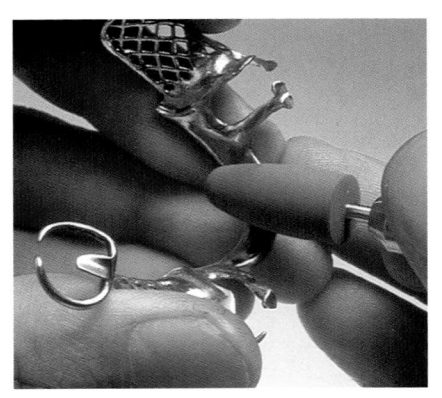

Image courtesy of Shofu Dental Corporation, www.shofu.com

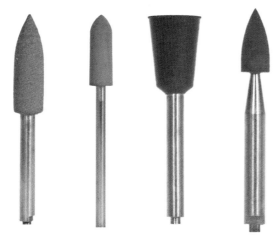

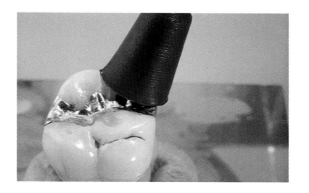

Images courtesy of Shofu Dental Corporation, www.shofu.com

PROPHY CUP AND BRUSH

FUNCTION:	To remove plaque and stain from coronal surfaces
FEATURES:	Latch or screw shank
	Brush—flat or pointed; black or white, soft or firm
	Cup—ribbed or webbed, soft or firm, rubber or latex-free
TRAY SET-UP:	Prophylaxis

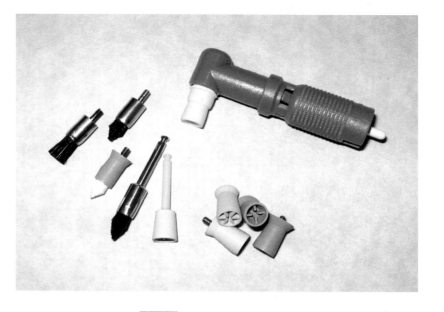

201

BUR HOLDER/BLOCK/CADDY

FUNCTION: Holds burs on tray set-up for easy viewing and retrieval

FEATURES: Different designs for varying number of burs and for different shank types

Some have movable bar that hold burs in place during ultrasonic cleaning and sterilization

May be magnetic to hold burs in place

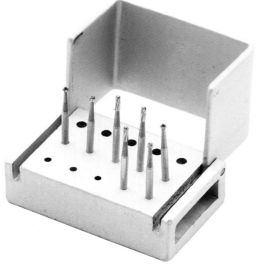

Images courtesy of Miltex, www.miltex.com

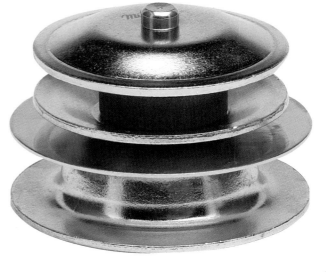

End Chapter 7

Impression Instruments and Equipment

ALGINATE SPATULA

FUNCTION: To mix alginate in a flexible bowl

TRAY SET-UP: Crown and bridge preparation; preliminary appointment for partial and complete dentures; orthodontic—initial records and final band removal; and initial appointment for fabrication of study models, bleaching trays, night guards, or other appliances

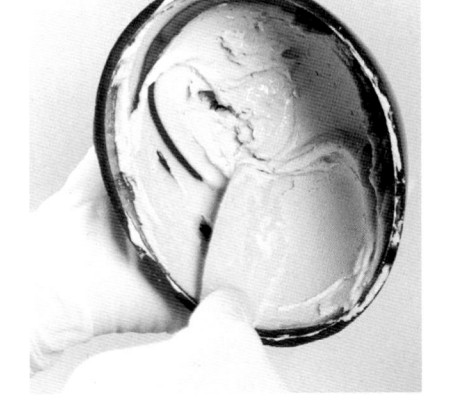

Reprinted with permission from Gladwin MA, Bagby M. Clinical aspects of dental materials: theory, practice, and cases. 3rd ed. Baltimore, MD: Lippincott Williams & Wilkins, 2008.

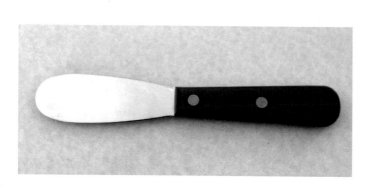

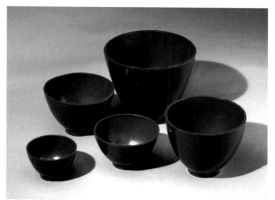

Image courtesy of Coltene Whaledent, www.coltene.com

ALGINATOR

FUNCTION: Automated mixer for mixing alginate and plaster

FEATURES: Attached bowl spins on base as alginate spatula is firmly held against the side of the bowl

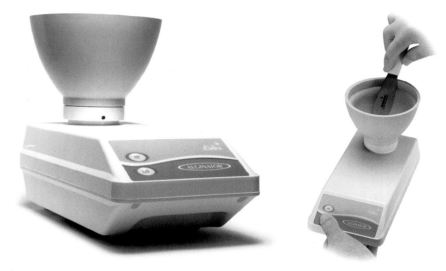

Images courtesy of Dux Dental, www.duxdental.com

IMPRESSION TRAYS

FUNCTION: To hold and carry impression materials to the mouth for obtaining a replica of the teeth and oral structures

FEATURES: Various sizes to fit all patients

Regular, edentulous, and pediatric

Metal and plastic; solid and perforated

Designs: full-arch, quadrant and anterior; maxillary, mandibular, and dual arch

CLINICAL APPLICATION: Double arch impression trays (Triple Tray®, Check-Bite™, 3-Way™, and others) are used for crown and bridge impressions and perform multiple functions with one tray. The design allows for a maxillary, mandibular, and bite registration all in one impression.

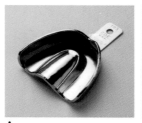 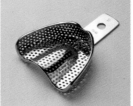 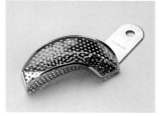

A

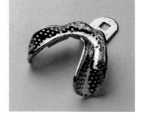

B

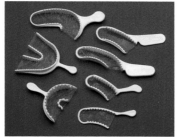

C

(A) Regular solid and perforated impression trays and (B) edentulous perforated impression trays courtesy of GC America, www.gcamerica.com; (C) assorted Triple Trays courtesy of Premier Dental Products, www.premusa.com

IMPRESSION PASTE SPATULA

FUNCTION: To mix elastomeric impression materials (vinyl polysiloxane, polyethers, rubber base/polysulfide, silicone, zinc oxide eugenol) and bite registration materials on paper pad

TRAY SET-UP: Crown and bridge preparation; partial and complete denture final impressions

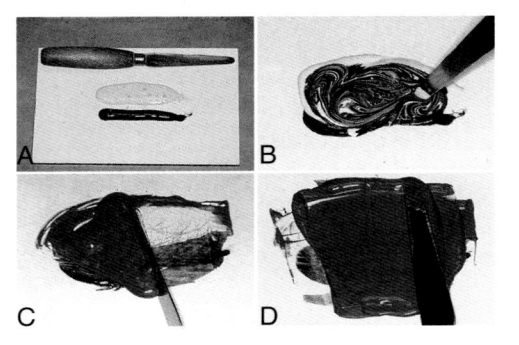

Reprinted with permission from Gladwin MA, Bagby M. Clinical aspects of dental materials: theory, practice, and cases. 3rd ed. Baltimore, MD: Lippincott Williams & Wilkins, 2008.

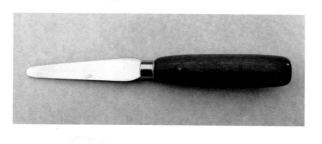

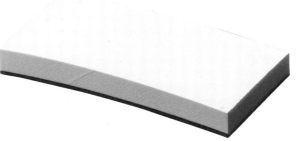

Image courtesy of Miltex, www.miltex.com

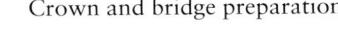

IMPRESSION MATERIAL SYRINGE

FUNCTION: To carry elastomeric impression materials to the mouth and to eject the material around the prepared tooth/teeth

TRAY SET-UP: Crown and bridge preparation

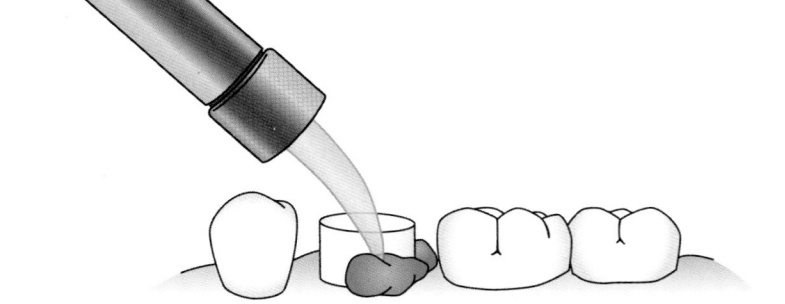

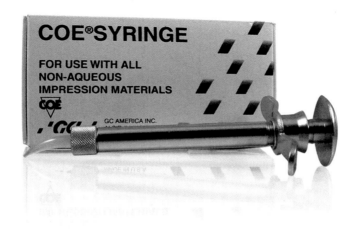

Image courtesy of GC America, www.gcamerica.com

CARTRIDGE DISPENSER

> **FUNCTION:** To mix and dispense impression materials and bite registration materials that are supplied in cartridges
>
> **FEATURES:** Dispensing "gun" style
>
> Used with specially designed mixing tips
>
> Dispenses on/in impression tray or impression syringe, or directly onto prepared tooth

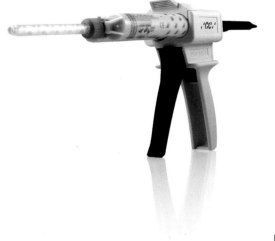

Reprinted with permission from Gladwin MA, Bagby M. Clinical aspects of dental materials: theory, practice, and cases. 3rd ed. Baltimore, MD: Lippincott Williams & Wilkins, 2008.

AUTOMIXER

FUNCTION: To mix and dispense vinyl polysiloxane and polyether impression materials that are supplied in large foil pouches or polybags

FEATURES: Countertop equipment

Dispenses on/in mixing pad, impression tray, or impression syringe

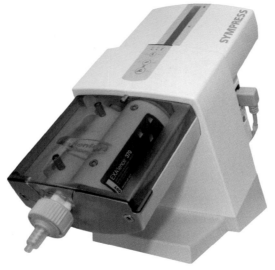

Image courtesy of GC America, www.gcamerica.com

End Chapter 8

PLASTER SPATULA

FUNCTION: To mix gypsum products (plaster, stone, investment) with water in a bowl

FEATURES: Stainless steel blade with wooden handle

Narrower blade than alginate spatula

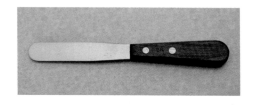

223

VIBRATOR

FUNCTION: To remove air in gypsum mixes and reduce voids in dental casts

FEATURES: Vibrating rubber coated platform
Three speeds

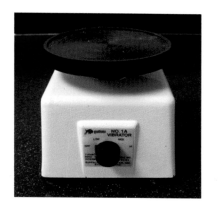

LAB KNIFE

FUNCTION: To trim plaster and stone on dental casts; compound and wax

FEATURES: Steel blades with wooden handle

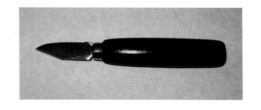

MODEL TRIMMER

FUNCTION: To grind and shape all types of dental models

FEATURES: Rotating carborundum wheel

Adjustable water supply to reduce dust, facilitate cutting, and clean wheel

Adjustable work table

Reprinted with permission from Gladwin MA, Bagby M. Clinical aspects of dental materials: theory, practice, and cases. 3rd ed. Baltimore, MD: Lippincott Williams & Wilkins, 2008.

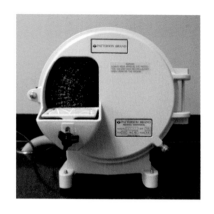

Laboratory
9

VACUUM FORMING UNIT

FUNCTION: To heat and soften thermo-plastic sheets for vacuum forming on dental cast. Used for fabrication of bleaching trays, mouth guards, night guards, splints, custom trays, and base plates.

FEATURES: Small electric equipment with heat source and vacuum

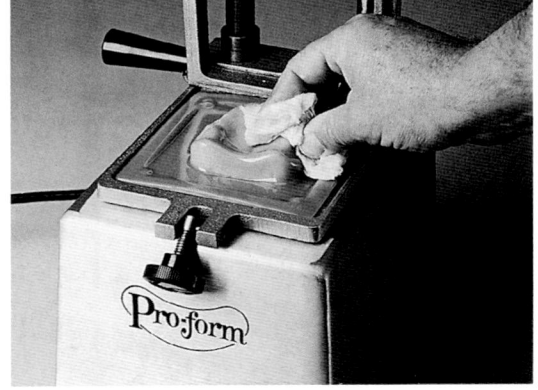

Reprinted with permission from Gladwin MA, Bagby M. Clinical aspects of dental materials: theory, practice, and cases. 3rd ed. Baltimore, MD: Lippincott Williams & Wilkins, 2008.

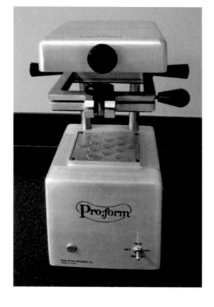

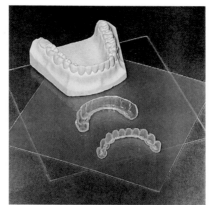

Reprinted with permission from Gladwin MA, Bagby M. Clinical aspects of dental materials: theory, practice, and cases. 3rd ed. Baltimore, MD: Lippincott Williams & Wilkins, 2008.

Laboratory
9

SCALLOPING SCISSORS

FUNCTION: To cut and scallop gingival edge of bleaching trays

FEATURES: Serrated blades

Spring handle

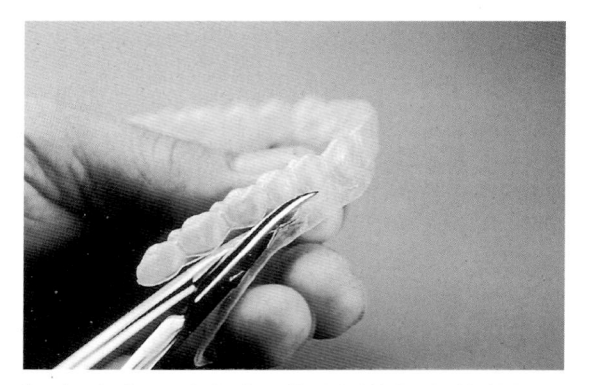

Reprinted with permission from Gladwin MA, Bagby M. Clinical aspects of dental materials: theory, practice, and cases. 3rd ed. Baltimore, MD: Lippincott Williams & Wilkins, 2008.

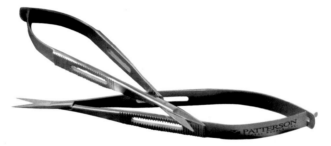

Image courtesy of Patterson Dental, www.pattersondental.com

233

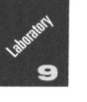

BOLEY GAUGE

FUNCTION: Metric rule (caliper) to measure length and diameter of teeth, oral structures, prosthetic appliances, and root canal instruments

TRAY SET-UP: Root canal, bite registration and wax try-in for removable dentures, cosmetic procedures

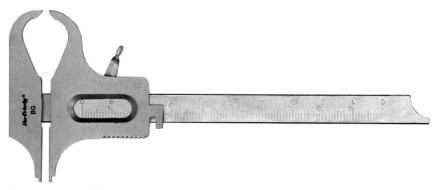

Image courtesy of Hu-Friedy, www.hu-friedy.com

235

Laboratory
9

7A WAX SPATULA

FUNCTION:	To manipulate wax during denture and crown fabrication procedures
FEATURES:	Double ended with one round, blunted end, and one pointed end
	Similar in appearance to a small periosteal elevator
TRAY SET-UP:	Removable denture bite registration and wax try-in
	Many laboratory uses

Image courtesy of Hu-Friedy, www.hu-friedy.com

ROACH WAX CARVER

FUNCTION:	To manipulate wax during denture and crown fabrication procedures
FEATURES:	Double ended with one spear-shaped end and one with a concave area for melting wax
TRAY SET-UP:	Removable denture bite registration and wax try-in
	Many laboratory uses

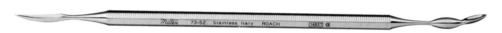

Image courtesy of Miltex, www.miltex.com

Laboratory 9

ARTICULATOR

FUNCTION: Simulates patient's occlusion and jaw movements for fabrication of crowns, bridges, and dentures

FEATURES: Mechanical device holds working casts

Metal or plastic

Various styles and sizes

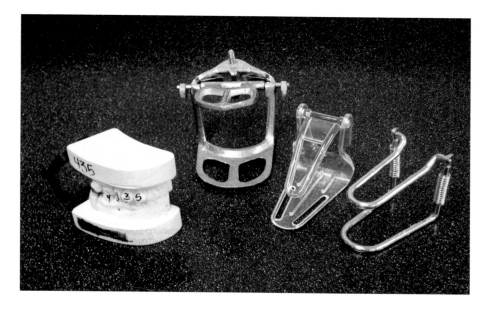

241

TRIAD® CURING UNIT

FUNCTION: Light cures TRIAD VLC material for fabricating custom trays, orthodontic appliances, provisional crowns and bridges, and denture repairs and relines

FEATURES: Curing chamber with rotating platform

Tungsten halogen light source

Cures light activated materials with visible light

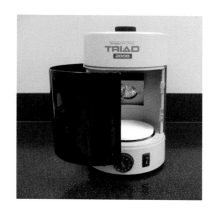

End Chapter 9

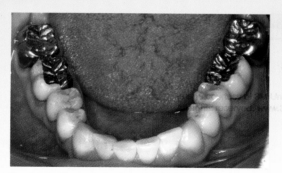

Reprinted with permission from Scheid RC. Woelfel's dental anatomy: its relevance to dentistry, 7th ed. Philadelphia: Lippincott Williams & Wilkins, 2007.

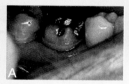

A

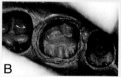

B

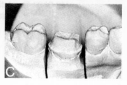

C

Reprinted with permission from Gladwin MA, Bagby M. Clinical aspects of dental materials: theory, practice, and cases. 3rd ed. Baltimore, MD: Lippincott Williams & Wilkins, 2008.

CROWN AND COLLAR SCISSORS

FUNCTION: To trim the gingival margins of temporary crowns

FEATURES: Straight or curved beaks

Also known as crown and bridge scissors

TRAY SET-UP: Crown preparation

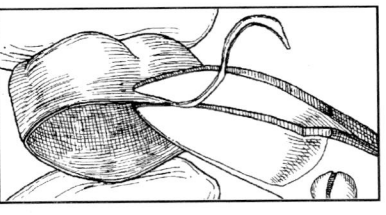

Image courtesy of University of Kentucky
(570 m-16a)

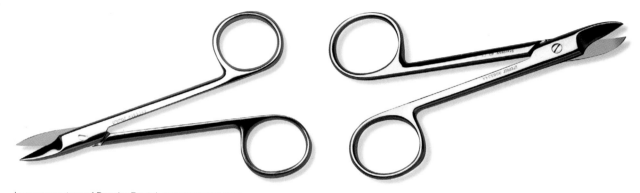

Images courtesy of Premier Dental, www.premusa.com

CONTOURING PLIERS

FUNCTION: To shape/crimp gingival edge of temporary crown for better adaptation

FEATURES: Common designs are the "bird beak" and "ball and socket"

TRAY SET-UP: Crown preparation

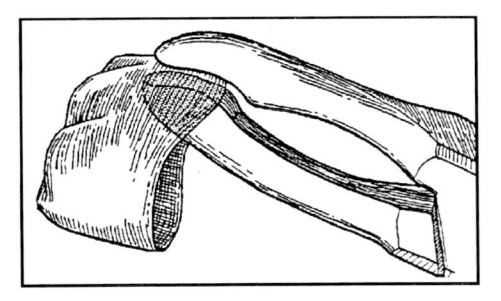

Image courtesy of University of Kentucky (570m-13)

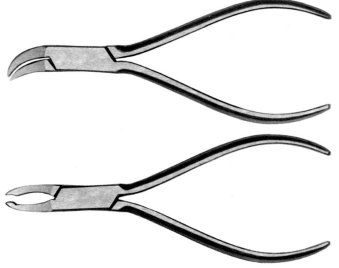

Images courtesy of Hu-Friedy, www.hu-friedy.com

CORD PACKERS

FUNCTION: To place retraction cord in gingival sulcus to control bleeding and to achieve gingival retraction during crown preparation and final impression

TRAY SET-UP: Crown and bridge preparation

VARIETIES: Serrated and nonserrated edges of blade

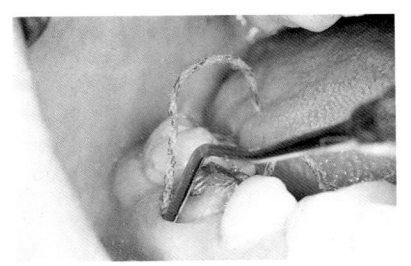

Image courtesy of Hu-Friedy,
www.hu-friedy.com

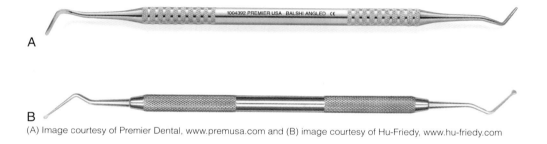

A

B

(A) Image courtesy of Premier Dental, www.premusa.com and (B) image courtesy of Hu-Friedy, www.hu-friedy.com

Crown
& Bridge
10

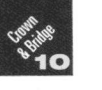

CEMENT SPATULA

FUNCTION: To mix dental cements for restorations, bases, or luting

FEATURES: Made of rigid or flexible metal, agate, and plastic

TRAY SET-UP: Restorative, crown and bridge preparation, crown and bridge seating

Image courtesy of Premier Dental, www.premusa.com

CROWN REMOVERS

FUNCTION: To remove temporary or permanent crowns

FEATURES: Morrel crown remover tip fits along cervical edge of crown. Barrel on the instrument shaft is moved up and down creating a pulling motion on the crown.

Other crown removers similar in appearance to a hemostat

TRAY SET-UP: Crown and bridge seating and cementing

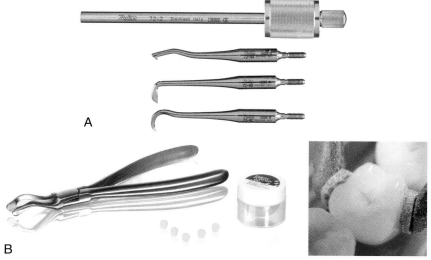

A

B

(A) Image courtesy of Miltex, www.miltex.com and (B) images courtesy of GC America, www.gcamerica.com

ACCU-PLACER

FUNCTION: Used with Accu-Dot® tape to hold and place veneers and inlays for bonding

TRAY SET-UP: Inlay and veneer bonding

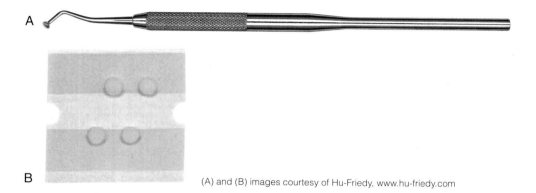

A

B

(A) and (B) images courtesy of Hu-Friedy, www.hu-friedy.com

CAD/CAM SYSTEMS

FUNCTION: To design and fabricate dental restorations (crowns, inlays, onlays, veneers) with ceramic and resin based materials in one appointment.

FEATURES: All CAD/CAM systems have three functional components: intraoral digital scanning device to record data about the tooth preparation, adjacent teeth and occluding teeth

CAD component to design a virtual model of the restoration

CAM component to fabricate, "mill" the restoration from a ceramic or composite resin block[1]

Current in-office systems are the CEREC (Sirona) and E4D (D4D Technologies)

CLINICAL APPLICATION: With these systems, a dentist can prepare, design, fabricate, and seat an indirect restoration in one appointment. This eliminates taking impressions and fabricating temporary crowns. However, the CAD/CAM system has a very high initial investment cost.

REFERENCE

Strub JR, Rekow D, Witkowski S. Computer-aided design and fabrication of dental restorations. *J Am Dent Assoc* 2006;137(9):1289–1296.

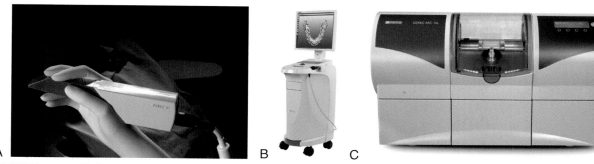

(A) CEREC camera, (B) CEREC acquisition unit, and (C) CEREC milling unit images courtesy of Sirona Dental Systems, www.sirona.com

CROWN AND BRIDGE PREPARATION SET-UP

PURPOSE: To provide instrumentation for preparing the tooth to support and retain an artificial crown, for making an impression of the tooth preparation, and for fabricating temporary coverage for the prepared tooth.

1. Basic set-up
2. Local anesthesia set-up
3. Floss
4. Diamonds and burs
5. Handpieces (high and low speed)
6. Spoon excavator
7. Cord packing instrument
8. Plastic instrument
9. Scaler
10. Crown and collar scissors
11. Articulating paper forceps
12. Temporary crowns
13. Contouring pliers
14. Mixing pad
15. Impression material
16. Impression tray
17. Impression paste spatula
18. Impression paste syringe
19. Temporary cement

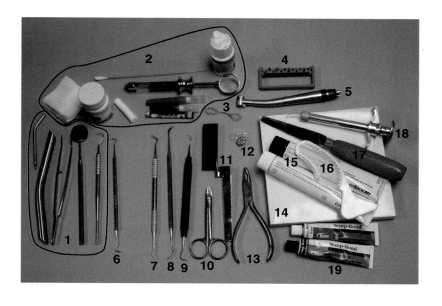

CROWN AND BRIDGE CEMENTATION SET-UP

PURPOSE: To provide instrumentation for removing the temporary coverage, adjusting fit and occlusion of permanent crown or bridge, and permanently cementing or bonding the restoration to the prepared tooth/teeth.

1. Basic set-up
2. Local anesthesia set-up
3. Crown remover
4. Towel clamp
5. Floss
6. Diamonds and burs
7. Handpieces (high and low speed)
8. Spoon excavator
9. Plastic instrument
10. Scaler
11. Bite stick
12. Articulating paper forceps
13. Cement spatula
14. Permanent cement
15. Mixing pad

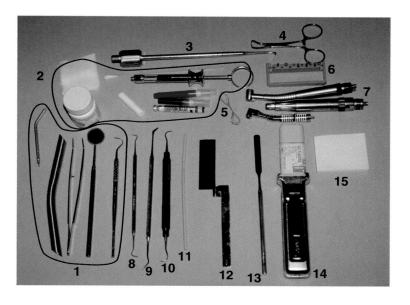

Crown
& Bridge
10

End Chapter 10

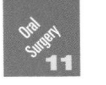
PERIOSTEAL ELEVATOR—MOLT

FUNCTION: To detach the periosteum from bone following an incision or to detach the gingival tissues from around the neck of the tooth prior to placement of extraction forceps

FEATURES: Double ended with one round, blunted end and one pointed end

TRAY SET-UP: Used for most surgical procedures: extractions, gingivoplasty, alveoplasty, cyst removal

CLINICAL APPLICATION: 7A wax spatula or a Woodson #1 plastic instrument is sometimes used if a smaller periosteal elevator is desired

Image courtesy of Hu-Friedy, www.hu-friedy.com

267

Oral Surgery
11

STRAIGHT ELEVATORS

FUNCTION: To loosen tooth or root from bony socket prior to placement of the extraction forceps

FEATURES: Straight handle and working end

Single rounded working end in several sizes

Often referred to by number—common sizes: 1, 34, 301

TRAY SET-UP: Tooth and root extraction

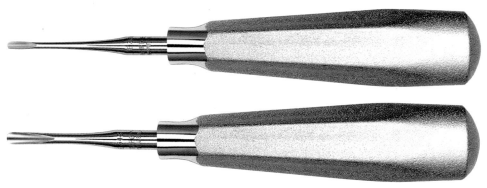

Images courtesy of Hu-Friedy, www.hu-friedy.com

269

ANGULAR ELEVATORS—CRYER

FUNCTION: To loosen tooth or root from bony socket prior to placement of the extraction forceps

FEATURES: Handles may be either large and straight or T-bar/crossbar design

Pointed working end in several sizes

Paired, right and left

Also called a "flag" elevator

Other common designs: Potts and Crane

TRAY SET-UP: Tooth and root extraction, impaction

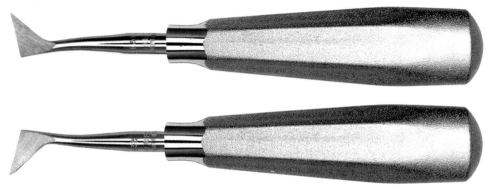

Images courtesy of Hu-Friedy, www.hu-friedy.com

271

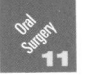

ANGULAR ELEVATORS—POTTS

FUNCTION: To loosen tooth or root from bony socket prior to placement of the extraction forceps

FEATURES: Handles may be either large and straight or T-bar/crossbar design

Rounded working end in several sizes

Paired, right and left

Other common designs: Cryer and Crane

TRAY SET-UP: Tooth and root extraction, impaction

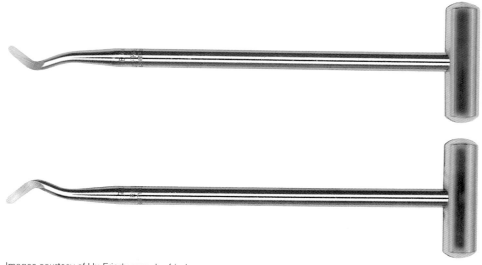

Images courtesy of Hu-Friedy, www.hu-friedy.com

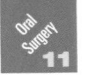

ANGULAR ELEVATORS—CRANE

FUNCTION: To loosen tooth or root from bony socket prior to placement of the extraction forceps

FEATURES: Large straight handle

Nonpaired, universal

Other common designs: Cryer and Potts

TRAY SET-UP: Tooth and root extraction, impaction

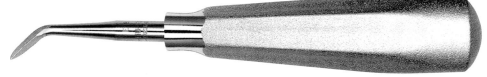

Image courtesy of Hu-Friedy, www.hu-friedy.com

275

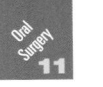
ROOT TIP PICKS—ANGLED

FUNCTION: To loosen small root fragments from bony socket

FEATURES: Small elevator with thin, pointed, angled working end
Single or double ended

TRAY SET-UP: Tooth and root extraction, impaction

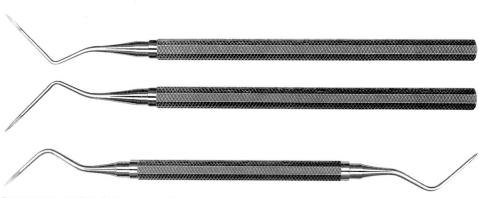

Images courtesy of Hu-Friedy, www.hu-friedy.com

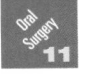

ROOT TIP PICKS—STRAIGHT

FUNCTION: To loosen small root fragments from bony socket

FEATURES: Small elevator with thin, pointed, straight working end
Single or double ended

TRAY SET-UP: Tooth and root extraction, impaction

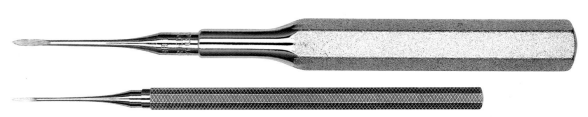

Image courtesy of Hu-Friedy, www.hu-friedy.com

SURGICAL CURETTES—DOUBLE ENDED/ANGULAR

FUNCTION: To remove tissue or debris from bony sockets

FEATURES: Spoon-shaped scraping instrument
Usually double ended and angular in several sizes

TRAY SET-UP: Extraction, impaction, and cyst removal

CLINICAL APPLICATION: Used following tooth extraction to ensure removal of debris and diseased tissue

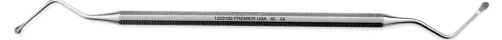

Image courtesy of Premier Dental Products, www.premusa.com

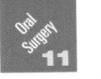

SURGICAL CURETTES—MOLT

FUNCTION: To remove tissue or debris from bony sockets

FEATURES: Single rounded working end with larger diameter handle

TRAY SET-UP: Extraction, impaction, cyst removal

CLINICAL APPLICATION: Molt #1 (pictured) also used to retract tissue flaps following incision

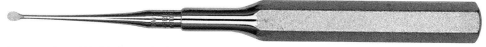

Image courtesy of Hu-Friedy, www.hu-friedy.com

283

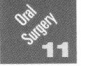

HEMOSTATS

FUNCTION: To securely hold small items, clamp blood vessels, and remove small pieces of tooth or bone

FEATURES: Angled or straight with locking, scissor-like handles

Common names: Mosquito, Kelly

Available in 4¾″, 5½″, 6¼″, and 7½″

TRAY SET-UP: Almost all surgical set-ups

CLINICAL APLICATION: Ratchet-type handles require some practice to open and close smoothly

Very versatile instrument used in all areas of dentistry

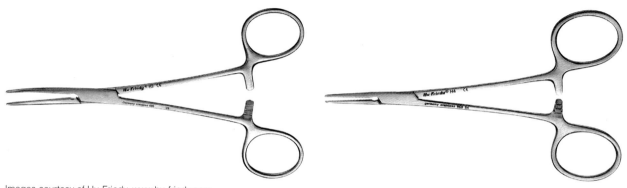

Images courtesy of Hu-Friedy, www.hu-friedy.com

Oral
Surgery
11

NEEDLE HOLDERS

FUNCTION:	To hold suture needle
FEATURES:	Similar to hemostat but with a concave area on inside of each beak to allow for curve of suture needle
TRAY SET-UP:	Any surgical procedure involving an incision will require placement of sutures
CLINICAL APPLICATION:	To avoid needle breakage, place the needle holder on the needle just beyond the suture attachment point and at right angles to the curve of the needle

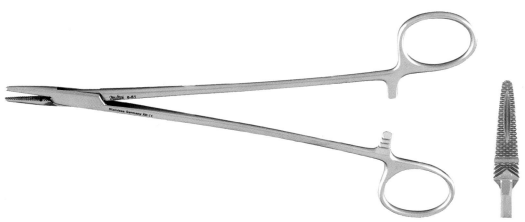

Images courtesy of Miltex, www.miltex.com

287

SUTURE

FUNCTION:	To close incision site
	"Stitches" hold tissues in place during healing
FEATURES:	Suture material attached to sterile stainless steel needle
	Different sizes and designs of needles
	Suture may be absorbable—plain or chromic gut, polyglycolic acid (PGA, Vicryl) or nonabsorbable—silk, polyester, nylon, polypropylene
	Sized by diameter of suture material: 3–0 (000), 4–0 (0000), 5–0 (00000) most common sizes used in dentistry (smaller number = larger diameter)
CLINICAL APPLICATION:	Nonabsorbable sutures usually removed at 7–10 days postsurgical visit
	Placed with needle holder or hemostat

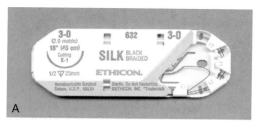

A

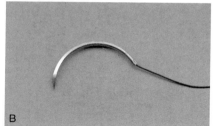

B

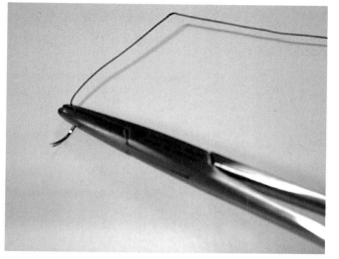

Oral Surgery
11

SCALPEL

FUNCTION:	To cut soft tissue—a surgical knife
FEATURES:	Often referred to as "Bard-Parker" or "BP"
	Individually sterile wrapped for single use
	Common blade sizes: #11 (a), #12 (b), #15 (c)
	Metal, sterilizable handle for replaceable blades (d)
	Disposable scalpel consisting of a plastic handle with attached blade (e)
TRAY SET-UP:	Most surgical set-ups: impaction, extraction, biopsy, frenectomy, gingivoplasty, alveoplasty, incision and drainage, and apicoectomy
CLINICAL APPLICATION:	For safety, blades are placed and removed from the metal handle with a hemostat or a specially designed scalpel blade remover
	Used blades should be disposed of in a sharps container

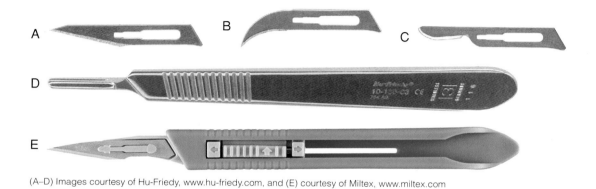

(A–D) Images courtesy of Hu-Friedy, www.hu-friedy.com, and (E) courtesy of Miltex, www.miltex.com

SCALPEL BLADE REMOVER

FUNCTION: To safely remove blade from scalpel handle

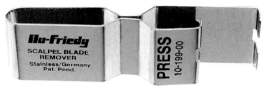

Image courtesy of Hu-Friedy, www.hu-friedy.com

Oral Surgery 11

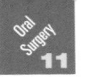

RONGEURS—SIDE-CUTTING

FUNCTION: To cut and contour bone—removes sharp edges of alveolar crest after extractions for better contour of alveolar ridge; removes exostoses

FEATURES: Scissor-type handle, cutting edges on side and top of beaks

TRAY SET-UP: Multiple extractions, alveolectomy/alveoplasty

CLINICAL APPLICATION: During use, bone will accumulate around cutting edges. Assistant should wipe working ends with 4 × 4 periodically to remove debris.

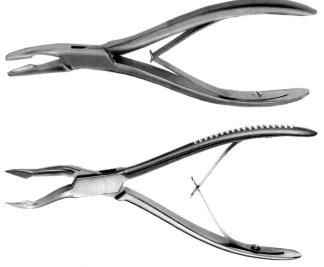

Oral
Surgery
11

RONGEURS—END-CUTTING

FUNCTION:	To cut and contour bone—removes sharp edges of alveolar crest after extractions for better contour of alveolar ridge; removes exostoses
FEATURES:	Scissor-type handle, cutting edges on top edge of beaks
TRAY SET-UP:	Multiple extractions, alveolectomy/alveoplasty
CLINICAL APPLICATION:	During use, bone will accumulate around cutting edges. Assistant should wipe working ends with 4 × 4 periodically to remove debris.

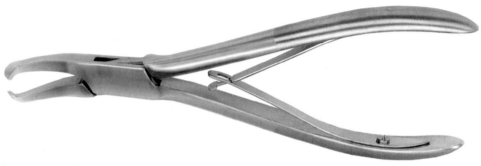

Image courtesy of Hu-Friedy, www.hu-friedy.com

Oral
Surgery
11

BONE CHISEL AND MALLET

FUNCTION: To remove bone for better contour of alveolar ridge; remove exostoses, i.e., tori

TRAY SET-UP: Tori removal, alveoplasty

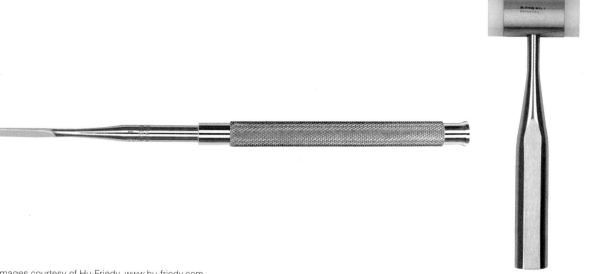

299

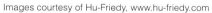

Oral
Surgery
11

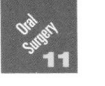

BONE FILE

FUNCTION: To smooth bone for better contour of alveolar ridge, often following use of rongeurs

FEATURES: Straight or curved working ends

Crosscut or straight cutting ridges

Double ended

TRAY SET-UP: Multiple extractions and impactions that require bone removal, tori removal, alveoplasty

CLINICAL APPLICATION: During use, bone will accumulate around cutting edges. Assistant should wipe working ends with 4 × 4 periodically to remove debris.

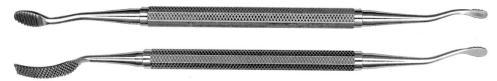

Images courtesy of Hu-Friedy, www.hu-friedy.com

TISSUE SCISSORS—DEAN

FUNCTION: To cut and remove excess or diseased soft tissue

Also used to cut sutures after knots are tied during suture placement

FEATURES: 6½"

Other common varieties of tissue scissors: Kelly, Iris

TRAY SET-UP: Gingivectomy/Gingivoplasty, frenectomy, multiple extractions

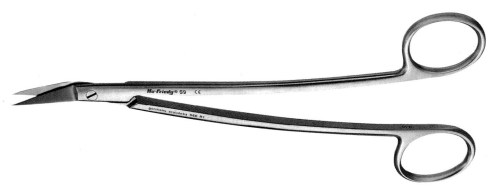

Image courtesy of Hu-Friedy, www.hu-friedy.com

303

Oral
Surgery
11

TISSUE SCISSORS—IRIS

FUNCTION: To cut and remove excess or diseased soft tissue

Also used to cut sutures after knots are tied during suture placement

FEATURES: Straight or curved, 4″ and 4½″

Other common varieties of tissue scissors: Dean, Kelly

TRAY SET-UP: Gingivectomy/gingivoplasty, frenectomy, multiple extractions

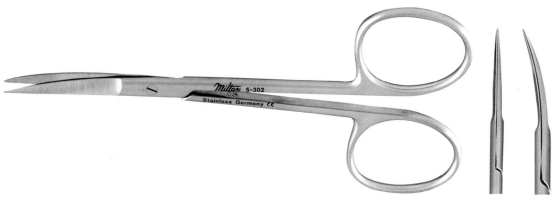

Images courtesy of Miltex, www.miltex.com

305

TISSUE SCISSORS—KELLY

FUNCTION: To cut and remove excess or diseased soft tissue

Also used to cut sutures after knots are tied during suture placement

FEATURES: Straight or curved, 6¼″ and 7″

Other common varieties of tissue scissors: Dean, Iris

TRAY SET-UP: Gingivectomy/gingivoplasty, frenectomy, multiple extractions

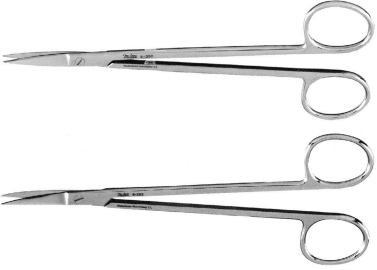

Images courtesy of Miltex, www.miltex.com

SUTURE SCISSORS

FUNCTION: To cut sutures for removal

FEATURES: One curved, hook-like tip to slip under suture

Holds suture away from tissue while cutting

$3\frac{1}{2}''$, $4\frac{1}{2}''$, $5\frac{1}{2}''$, and $6''$

TRAY SET-UP: Suture removal

CLINICAL APPLICATION: Suture removal often performed by the dental assistant. Wipe area clean with moistened 2×2, place curved scissor beak under suture near the knot, then grasp the knot with cotton plier or hemostat, and pull the suture out.

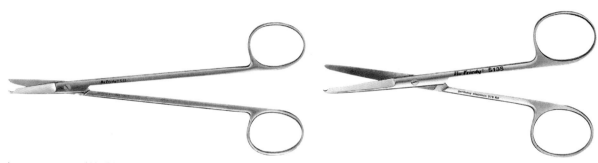

Images courtesy of Hu-Friedy, www.hu-friedy.com

309

TOWEL CLAMPS

FUNCTION:	To secure surgical drapes and to secure plastic and rubber tubing to drapes
FEATURES:	Sharp prong tips
	3½″ and 5¼″
	Additional use: Remove metal temporary crowns
TRAY SET-UP:	Any procedure when face and head are draped to isolate surgical area

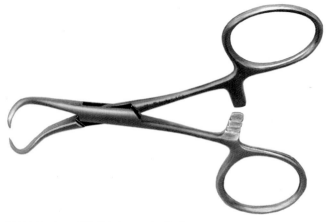

Image courtesy of Hu-Friedy, www.hu-friedy.com

Oral
Surgery
11

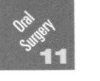
TISSUE RETRACTOR—AUSTIN

FUNCTION: To deflect and retract the periosteum from bone following an incision

FEATURES: L-shaped with one rounded end and one forked end

Other common designs: Seldin, Senn

TRAY SET-UP: All surgical procedures

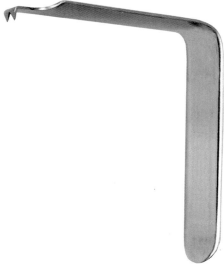

Image courtesy of Hu-Friedy, www.hu-friedy.com

Oral
Surgery
11

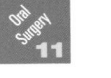

TISSUE RETRACTOR—SENN

FUNCTION:	To deflect and retract the periosteum from bone following an incision
FEATURES:	Double ended with one rounded and one forked end
	Other common designs: Austin, Seldin
TRAY SET-UP:	All surgical procedures

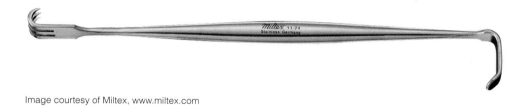

Image courtesy of Miltex, www.miltex.com

315

TISSUE RETRACTOR/PERIOSTEAL ELEVATOR—SELDIN

FUNCTION: To deflect and retract a tissue flap from bone following an incision

FEATURES: Double ended with round, blunted ends

TRAY SET-UP: Used for most surgical procedures: extractions, gingivoplasty, alveoplasty, cyst removal

Image courtesy of Hu-Friedy, www.hu-friedy.com

TONGUE AND CHEEK RETRACTOR—MINNESOTA

FUNCTION: To hold tongue and cheek away from surgical site

Other common designs: Shuman, Weider

TRAY SET-UP: All surgical procedures

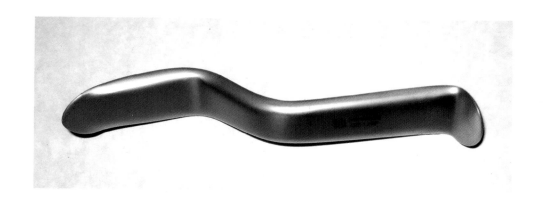

Oral
Surgery
11

TONGUE AND CHEEK RETRACTOR—SHUMAN

FUNCTION: To hold tongue and cheek away from surgical site

Other common designs: Minnesota, Weider

TRAY SET-UP: All surgical procedures

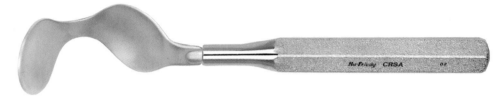

Image courtesy of Hu-Friedy, www.hu-friedy.com

TONGUE AND CHEEK RETRACTOR—WEIDER

FUNCTION: To hold tongue and cheek away from surgical site

Other common designs: Minnesota, Shuman

TRAY SET-UP: All surgical procedures

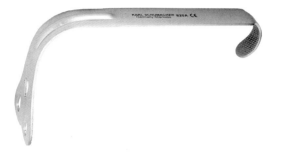

Image courtesy of Karl Schumacher Dental Instruments Company, Inc., www.karlschumacher.com

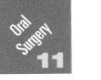
MOUTH PROP—BITE-BLOCK

FUNCTION: To keep mouth open with extensive procedures, sedated or disabled patients

FEATURES: Sterilizable rubber block in four sizes for children and adults
Other common design: mouth gag

TRAY SET-UP: Any procedure when patient may have difficulty keeping mouth open

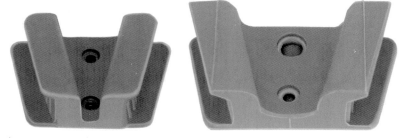

Images courtesy of Hu-Friedy, www.hu-friedy.com

Oral Surgery
11

MOUTH PROP—MOUTH GAG

FUNCTION: To keep mouth open with extensive procedures, sedated or disabled patients

FEATURES: Rachet design with rubber tips
Other common design: bite-block

TRAY SET-UP: Any procedure when patient may have difficulty keeping mouth open

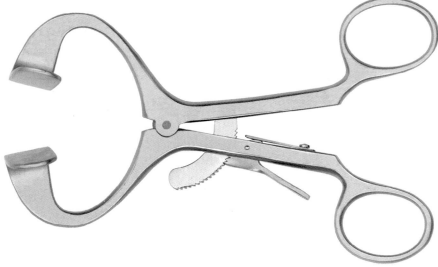

Image courtesy of Hu-Friedy, www.hu-friedy.com

SURGICAL ASPIRATING TIP—BYRD SELF-CLEANING

FUNCTION: To maintain a clear working field by removing saliva, blood, and debris

FEATURES: Built-in stylet to clear tip of bone or tooth fragments

Available in several diameters

Other common designs: Frazier, Cogswell

TRAY SET-UP: All surgical procedures

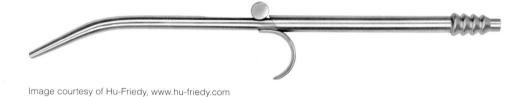

Image courtesy of Hu-Friedy, www.hu-friedy.com

Oral
Surgery
11

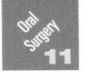

SURGICAL ASPIRATING TIP—COGSWELL

FUNCTION:	To maintain a clear working field by removing saliva, blood, and debris
FEATURES:	Vacuum relief hole controls suction by covering/uncovering the hole with fingertip
	Other common designs: Byrd, Frazier
TRAY SET-UP:	All surgical procedures
CLINICAL APPLICATION:	Tips are cleaned with long, flexible cleaning brushes

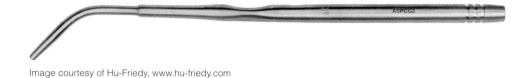

Image courtesy of Hu-Friedy, www.hu-friedy.com

331

SURGICAL ASPIRATING TIP—FRAZIER

FUNCTION:	To maintain a clear working field by removing saliva, blood, and debris
FEATURES:	Removable stylet to clear tip of bone or tooth fragments
	Vacuum relief hole controls suction by covering/uncovering the hole with fingertip
	Available in several diameters
	Other common designs: Byrd, Cogswell
TRAY SET-UP:	All surgical procedures

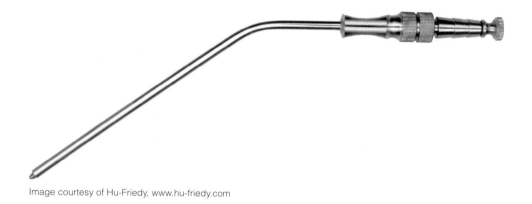

Image courtesy of Hu-Friedy, www.hu-friedy.com

Oral
Surgery
11

SURGICAL ASPIRATING TIP—YANKEUR TONSIL ASPIRATOR

FUNCTION: To suction throat when using general anesthesia

FEATURES: Angled with perforated ball-type end for suctioning throat

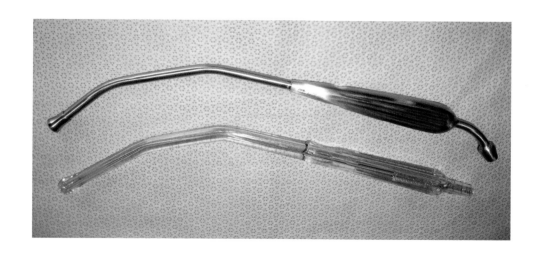

335

TISSUE PLIERS—ADSON

FUNCTION: To grasp and stabilize soft tissue flaps during suturing and reconstructive procedures such as gingival grafting

FEATURES: Similar in overall appearance to cotton pliers

Various serrated tips for securely grasping tissue flaps

TRAY SET-UP: Any surgical procedure requiring an incision and suturing

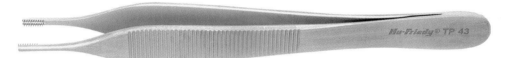

Image courtesy of Hu-Friedy, www.hu-friedy.com

337

TISSUE FORCEPS—ALLISON

FUNCTION: To grasp and stabilize soft tissue flaps during suturing and reconstructive procedures such as gingival grafting

FEATURES: Hemostat-type handles, serrated tips

TRAY SET-UP: Any surgical procedure requiring an incision and suturing

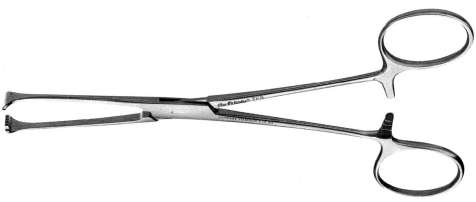

Image courtesy of Hu-Friedy, www.hu-friedy.com

339

EXTRACTION FORCEPS—#99 MAXILLARY ANTERIORS AND PREMOLARS

FUNCTION: To remove teeth from bony socket

FEATURES: Straight handle and beaks

Beaks designed to conform to facial and lingual root contour just apical to cervical line

Universal (both beaks same design-fit equally well on facial and lingual) for right and left quadrants

TRAY SET-UP: Extraction

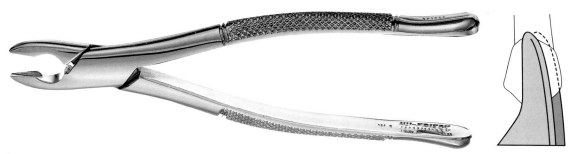

Images courtesy of Hu-Friedy, www.hu-friedy.com

EXTRACTION FORCEPS—#150 (CRYER) MAXILLARY ANTERIORS AND PREMOLARS

FUNCTION: To remove teeth from bony socket

FEATURES: Beaks designed to conform to facial and lingual root contour just apical to
cervical line

Universal (both beaks same design-fit equally well on facial and lingual) for right
and left quadrants

Maxillary counterpart to #151 Mandibular Cryer

TRAY SET-UP: Extraction

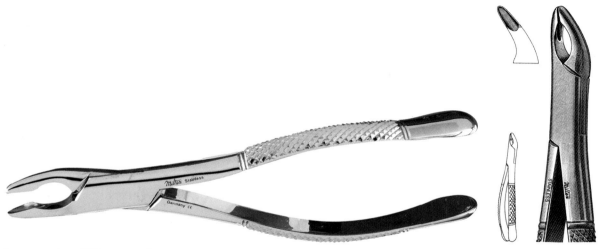

Images courtesy of Miltex, www.miltex.com

EXTRACTION FORCEPS—#18R MAXILLARY RIGHT FIRST AND SECOND MOLARS

FUNCTION: To remove teeth from bony socket

FEATURES: Each beak has different design to adapt to the maxillary molar roots that differ anatomically on the facial and lingual

Rounded beak contours to lingual root

Pointed beak contours to bifurcation of mesial–buccal and distal–buccal root #18R and #53R are essentially the same instrument except that #18R has one curved handle while both handles are straight on #53R

TRAY SET-UP: Extraction

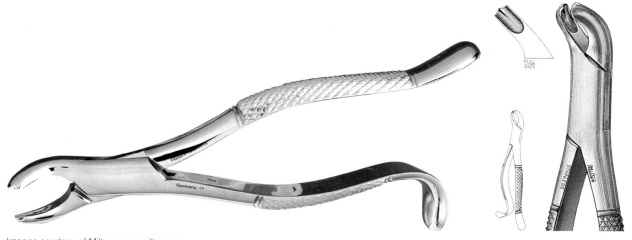

Images courtesy of Miltex, www.miltex.com

345

Oral Surgery 11

EXTRACTION FORCEPS—#18 L MAXILLARY LEFT FIRST AND SECOND MOLARS

FUNCTION: To remove teeth from bony socket

FEATURES: Each beak has different design to adapt to the maxillary molar roots that differ anatomically on the facial and lingual

Rounded beak contours to lingual root

Pointed beak contours to bifurcation of mesial–buccal and distal–buccal root #18L and #53L are essentially the same instrument except that #18L has one curved handle while both handles are straight on #53L

TRAY SET-UP: Extraction

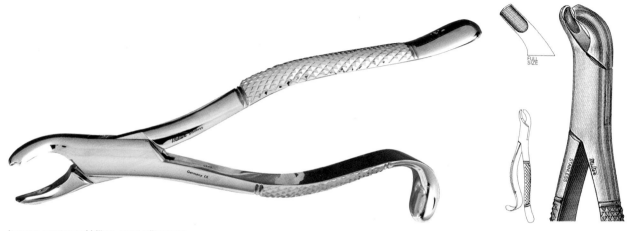

Images courtesy of Miltex, www.miltex.com

347

Oral Surgery
11

EXTRACTION FORCEPS—#53R MAXILLARY RIGHT FIRST AND SECOND MOLARS

FUNCTION: To remove teeth from bony socket

FEATURES: Bayonet design

Each beak has different design to adapt to the maxillary molar roots that differ anatomically on the facial and lingual

Rounded beak contours to lingual root

Pointed beak contours to bifurcation of mesial–buccal and distal–buccal roots #53R and #18R are essentially the same instrument except that #18R has one curved handle while both handles are straight on #53R

TRAY SET-UP: Extraction

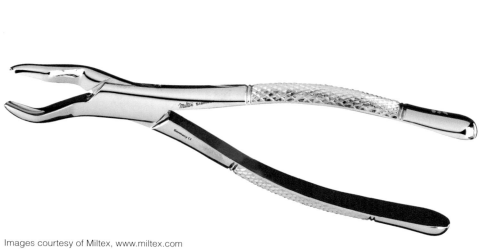

Images courtesy of Miltex, www.miltex.com

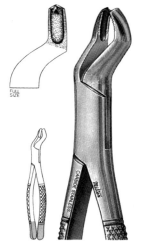

FULL
SIZE

CARBIDE STAINLESS

Miltex

349

Oral
Surgery
11

FUNCTION: To remove teeth from bony socket

FEATURES: Bayonet design

Each beak has different design to adapt to the maxillary molar roots that differ anatomically on the facial and lingual

Rounded beak contours to lingual root

Pointed beak contours to bifurcation of mesial–buccal and distal–buccal roots #53L and #18L are essentially the same instrument except that #18L has one curved handle while both handles are straight on #53L

TRAY SET-UP: Extraction

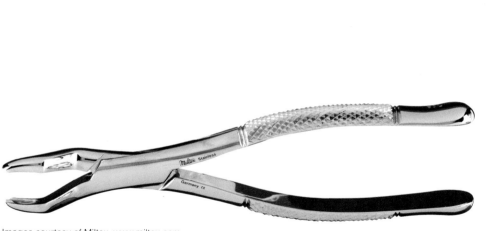

Images courtesy of Miltex, www.miltex.com

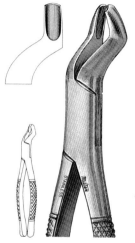

EXTRACTION FORCEPS—#88R MAXILLARY RIGHT FIRST AND SECOND MOLARS

FUNCTION: To remove teeth from bony socket

FEATURES: Bayonet design

Each beak has different design to adapt to the maxillary molar roots that differ anatomically on the facial and lingual

Beak with 1 projection contours to bifurcation of mesial–buccal and distal–buccal roots

Beak with two projections contours to lingual root

TRAY SET-UP: Extraction

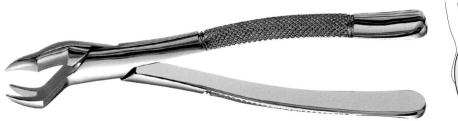
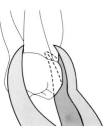

Images courtesy of Hu-Friedy, www.hu-friedy.com

353

FUNCTION: To remove teeth from bony socket

FEATURES: Bayonet design

Each beak has different design to adapt to the maxillary molar roots that differ anatomically on the facial and lingual

Beak with one projection contours to bifurcation of mesial–buccal and distal–buccal roots

Beak with two projections contours to lingual root

TRAY SET-UP: Extraction

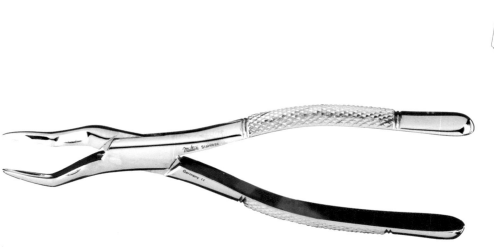

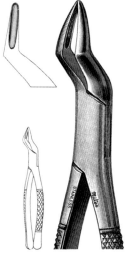

Images courtesy of Miltex, www.miltex.com

EXTRACTION FORCEPS—#74 MANDIBULAR ROOT TIPS

FUNCTION: To remove tooth fragments and root tips from bony socket

FEATURES: Bird beak design

Universal (both beaks same design-fit equally well on facial and lingual) for right and left quadrants

TRAY SET-UP: Extraction

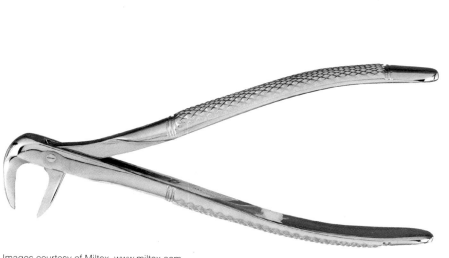
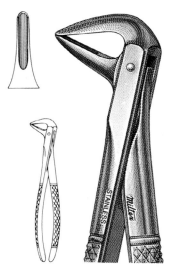

Images courtesy of Miltex, www.miltex.com

363

EXTRACTION FORCEPS—#101 ALL DECIDUOUS TEETH AND MANDIBULAR ANTERIORS

FUNCTION: To remove teeth from bony socket

FEATURES: Smaller overall

Beaks designed to conform to facial and lingual root contour just apical to cervical line

Universal (both beaks same design-fit equally well on facial and lingual) for right and left quadrants

TRAY SET-UP: Extraction

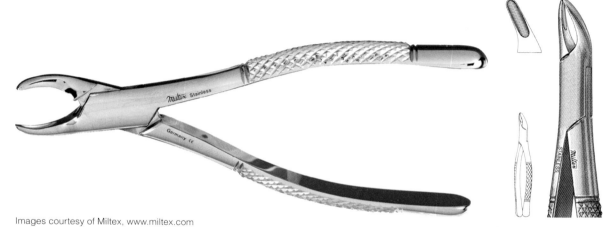

Images courtesy of Miltex, www.miltex.com

365

EXTRACTION FORCEPS—#103 MANDIBULAR ANTERIORS AND PREMOLARS

FUNCTION: To remove teeth from bony socket

FEATURES: Straight handle and beaks

Beaks designed to conform to facial and lingual root contour just apical to cervical line

Universal (both beaks same design-fit equally well on facial and lingual) for right and left quadrants

TRAY SET-UP: Extraction

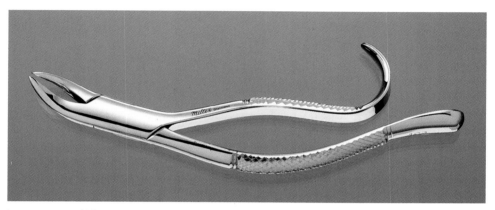

Image courtesy of Miltex, www.miltex.com

367

EXTRACTION FORCEPS—#151 (CRYER) MANDIBULAR ANTERIORS AND PREMOLARS

FUNCTION: To remove teeth from bony socket

FEATURES: Beaks designed to conform to facial and lingual root contour just apical to cervical line

Universal (both beaks same design-fit equally well on facial and lingual) for right and left quadrants

Mandibular counterpart to #150 Maxillary Cryer

TRAY SET-UP: Extraction

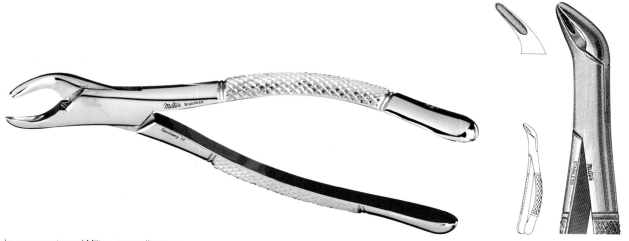

Oral Surgery
11

EXTRACTION FORCEPS—#15 MANDIBULAR FIRST AND SECOND MOLARS

FUNCTION: To remove teeth from bony socket

FEATURES: Beaks designed to conform to facial and lingual root contour just apical to cervical line

Universal (both beaks same design-fit equally well on facial and lingual) for right and left quadrants

Pointed beaks contour to bifurcation area of mesial and distal root

#15 and #17 are essentially the same instrument except that #15 has one curved handle while both handles are straight on #17

TRAY SET-UP: Extraction

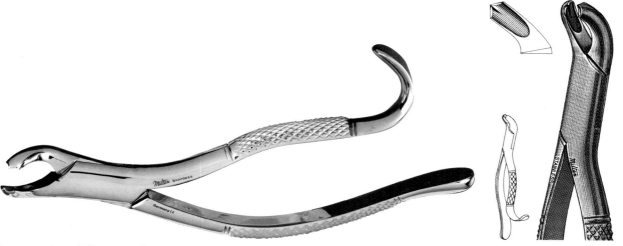

Images courtesy of Miltex, www.miltex.com

EXTRACTION FORCEPS—#17 MANDIBULAR FIRST AND SECOND MOLARS

FUNCTION: To remove teeth from bony socket

FEATURES: Beaks designed to conform to facial and lingual root contour just apical to cervical line

Universal (both beaks same design-fit equally well on facial and lingual) for right and left quadrants

Pointed beaks contour to bifurcation area of mesial and distal root

#17 and #15 are essentially the same instrument except that #15 has one curved handle while both handles are straight on #17

TRAY SET-UP: Extraction

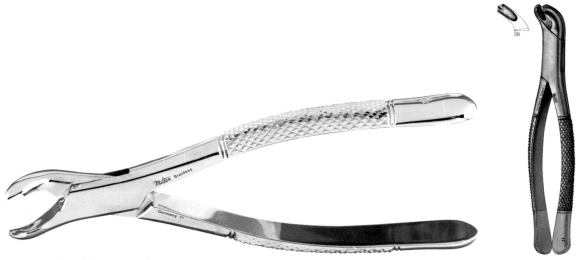

Images courtesy of Miltex, www.miltex.com

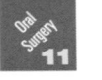

EXTRACTION FORCEPS—#16 MANDIBULAR FIRST AND SECOND MOLARS

FUNCTION: To remove teeth from bony socket

FEATURES: "Cowhorn" forceps

Beaks designed to conform to facial and lingual root contour just apical to cervical line

Universal (both beaks same design-fit equally well on facial and lingual) for right and left quadrants

Pointed beaks contour to bifurcation area of mesial and distal root

#16 and #23 are essentially the same instrument except that #16 has one curved handle while both handles are straight on #23

TRAY SET-UP: Extraction

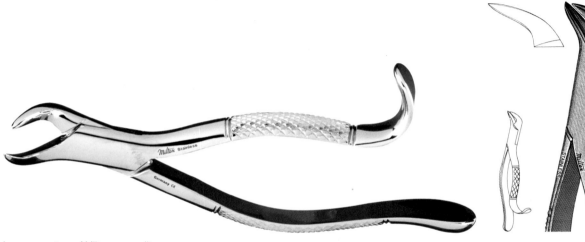

375

Oral
Surgery
11

EXTRACTION FORCEPS—#23 MANDIBULAR FIRST AND SECOND MOLARS

FUNCTION: To remove teeth from bony socket

FEATURES: "Cowhorn" forceps

Beaks designed to conform to facial and lingual root contour just apical to cervical line

Universal (both beaks same design-fit equally well on facial and lingual) for right and left quadrants

Pointed beaks contour to bifurcation area of mesial and distal root

#23 and #16 are essentially the same instrument except that #16 has one curved handle while both handles are straight on #23

TRAY SET-UP: Extraction

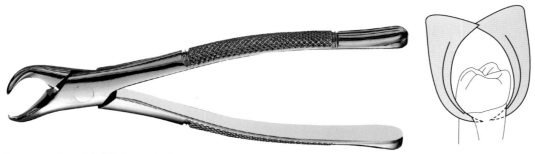

Images courtesy of Hu-Friedy, www.hu-friedy.com

377

EXTRACTION FORCEPS—#222 MANDIBULAR THIRD MOLARS

FUNCTION: To remove teeth from bony socket

FEATURES: Bayonet design

Beaks designed to conform to facial and lingual root contour just apical to cervical line

Universal (both beaks same design-fit equally well on facial and lingual) for right and left quadrants

TRAY SET-UP: Extraction

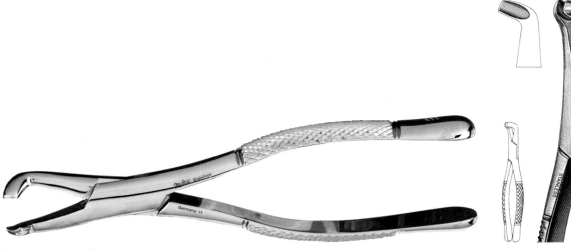

Images courtesy of Miltex, www.miltex.com

Oral
Surgery
11

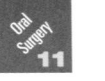

SURGICAL HANDPIECE

FUNCTION: To place implants, remove bone, section teeth

FEATURES: Holds sterile water and equipped with pump for oral irrigation
Both straight and contra angle handpiece designs
Variable speed and torque

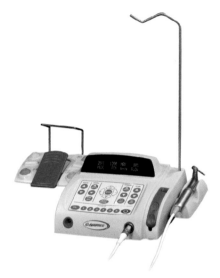

Image courtesy of Aseptico, www.aseptico.com

LASER (LIGHT AMPLIFICATION BY SIMULATED EMISSION OF RADIATION)

FUNCTION: To remove soft tissue with minimal discomfort and bleeding

Laser also has bacteriocidal effects for enhanced wound healing

APPLICATIONS: Frenectomy, excision of lesions, gingivoplasty, crown lengthening, root canal therapy

CLINICAL APPLICATION: Laser beam is hazardous to eyes and skin. Patient, operator, and assistant must wear special protective goggles and keep hands and body parts away from the beam. Nonshiny instruments should be used to avoid reflection of laser energy. Smoke plume forms as tissue is vaporized; use high volume evacuation during procedure.

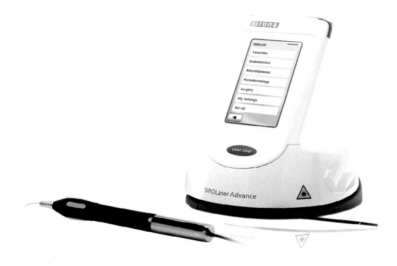

Image courtesy of Sirona Dental Systems, www.sirona.com

Oral Surgery 11

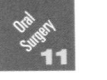

ENDOSSEOUS IMPLANT FIXTURE

FUNCTION: To provide a root form for replacement of missing teeth

FEATURES: Cylindrical, screw-shaped device
Made of titanium alloy
Embedded within the alveolar bone
Provides support for a dental crown, bridge, or denture

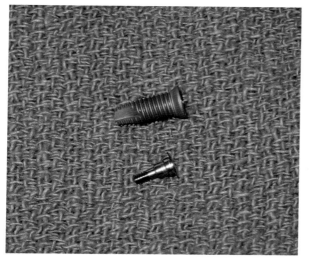

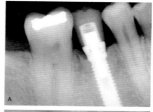

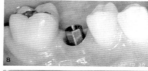

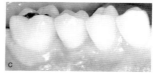

Photographs courtesy of Ed McGlumphy, D.D.S., M.S.,
Associate Professor, Ohio State University, College of Dentistry.

SURGICAL IMPLANT SITE PREPARATION KIT

FUNCTION: To remove and shape bone for placement of an implant fixture

FEATURES: Multiple "drill" shapes and sizes

CLINICAL APPLICATION: An incision is made and a tissue flap detached to expose the alveolar bone of the implant site. Next, a surgical handpiece is used with the implant site preparation kit to shape a hole for the implant fixture. The implant fixture is placed and covered with the soft tissue flap.

Reprinted with permission from Gladwin MA, Bagby M. Clinical aspects of dental materials: theory, practice, and cases. 3rd ed. Baltimore, MD: Lippincott Williams & Wilkins, 2008.

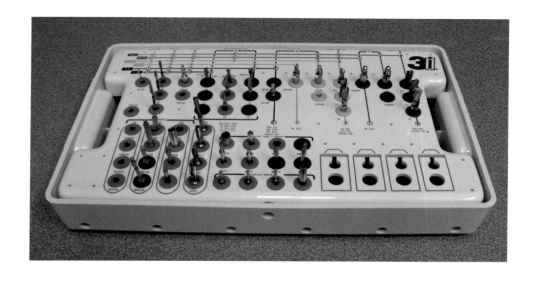

387

IMPLANT WRENCH/DRIVER

FUNCTION: To place implant screw or healing abutment on implant fixture

CLINICAL APPLICATION: The healing abutment extends above the oral mucosa. After the dental implant is stable and integrated with the bone, the top of the implant is exposed and the healing abutment is placed. The gingiva heals and grows around the abutment creating an esthetic gingival margin for the future implant crown.

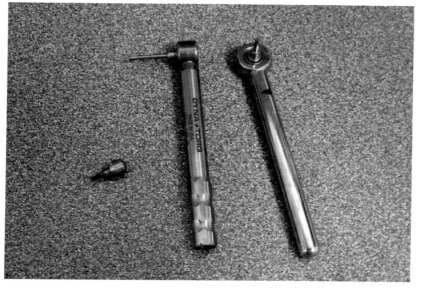

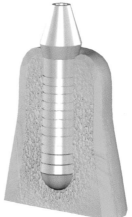

Oral
Surgery
11

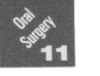

BASIC EXTRACTION SET-UP

PURPOSE: To provide instrumentation for surgical removal of tooth/teeth.

1. Local anesthesia syringe, needles, and cartridges
2. Sterile gauze
3. Surgical aspirating tip
4. Cotton pliers
5. Mouth mirror
6. Periosteal elevator
7. Straight elevators
8. Surgical curette
9. Hemostat
10. Extraction forceps (selected for specific tooth/teeth)

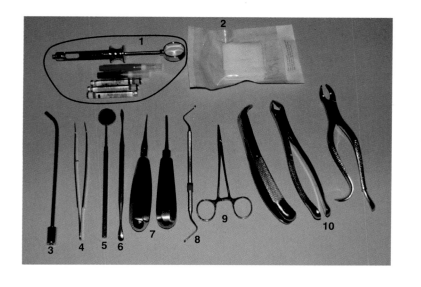

MULTIPLE EXTRACTION/ALVEOPLASTY/GINGIVOPLASTY SET-UP

PURPOSE: To provide instrumentation for surgically removing multiple teeth, reshaping bone and gingiva, and placing sutures.

1. Local anesthesia set-up
2. Tissue retractor
3. Scalpel(s)
4. Mouth prop
5. Sterile gauze
6. Surgical aspirating tip
7. Cotton pliers
8. Mouth mirror
9. Periosteal elevator
10. Straight elevators

11. Tissue retractor
12. Surgical curette
13. Bone file
14. Extraction forceps (selected for specific tooth/teeth)
15. Rongeur
16. Tissue scissor
17. Needle holder
18. Hemostat
19. Suture

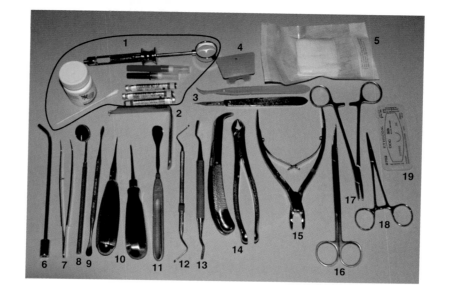

393

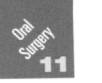

IMPACTION SET-UP

PURPOSE: To provide instrumentation for surgically removing impacted tooth. Often involves incision and bone removal.

1. Anesthetic syringe, needles, and cartridges
2. Mouth prop
3. Tissue retractor
4. Austin tissue retractor
5. Surgical bur
6. Hemostat
7. Surgical aspirating tip
8. Mouth mirror
9. Cotton pliers
10. Periosteal elevator
11. Straight elevator
12. Crane pick
13. Angular elevators
14. Root tip picks
15. Surgical curette
16. Molt curette
17. Bone file
18. Tissue scissor
19. Extraction forceps
20. Needle holder
21. Scalpel(s)
22. Suture

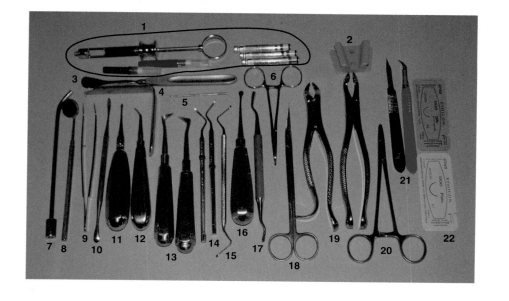

SUTURE REMOVAL SET-UP

1. Mouth mirror
2. Explorer
3. Suture removal scissors
4. Cotton pliers
5. Oral evacuator tip
6. Air/water syringe tip
7. 2 × 2 gauze

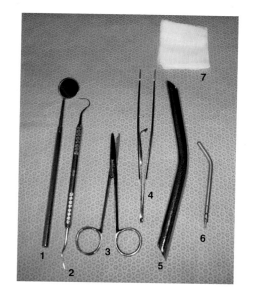

Oral
Surgery
11

End Chapter 11

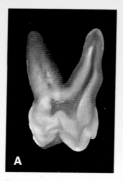
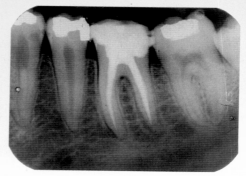

Reprinted with permission from Scheid RC. Woelfel's dental anatomy: its relevance to dentistry, 7th ed. Philadelphia: Lippincott Williams & Wilkins, 2007.

ENDO EXPLORERS

FUNCTION: To locate canal opening

TRAY SET-UP: Root canal

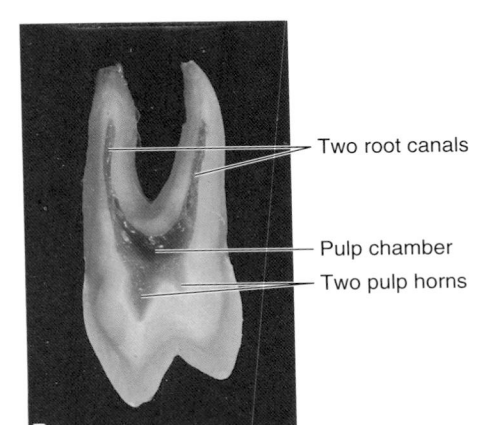

Two root canals

Pulp chamber

Two pulp horns

Reprinted with permission from Scheid RC. Woelfel's dental anatomy: its relevance to dentistry, 7th ed. Philadelphia: Lippincott Williams & Wilkins, 2007.

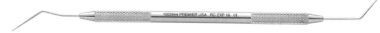

Image courtesy of Premier Dental Products, www.premusa.com

ENDO EXCAVATORS

FUNCTION: To remove pulp in pulp chamber; remove temporary filling and cotton pellets from chamber

TRAY SET-UP: Root canal, pulpotomy

Image courtesy of Premier Dental Products, www.premusa.com

ENDODONTIC DRILL

FUNCTION:	To open coronal access, enlarge the cervical portion of the canal, and prepare the canal entrance
FEATURES:	Latch-type rotary instrument
	Gates Glidden Drills and Peeso Drills/Reamers
TRAY SET-UP:	Root canal

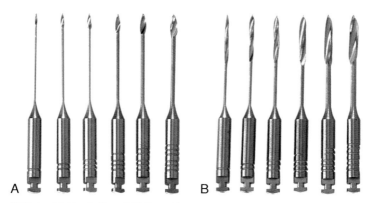

(A) Gates Glidden Drills and (B) Peeso Reamers courtesy of Miltex, www.miltex.com

Endodontic
12

BROACH

FUNCTION: To initially remove pulp from canal space

FEATURES: Stainless steel tips with fine barbs
DIAMETER SIZES: xxxfine—coarse

TRAY SET-UP: Root canal

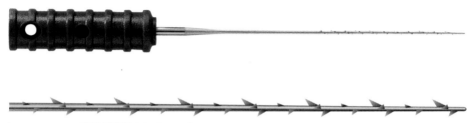

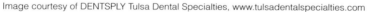

Image courtesy of DENTSPLY Tulsa Dental Specialties, www.tulsadentalspecialties.com

407

REAMER

FUNCTION: To remove pulp from canals; enlarge and shape canals for restorative materials

FEATURES: Stainless steel

TIP SIZE (DIAMETER): 6, 8, 10, 15, 20, 25, 30, 35, 40, 45, 50, 55, 60, 70, 80, 90–110, 120–140

LENGTHS: 21, 25, and 31 mm

Hand or handpiece driven

TRAY SET-UP: Root canal

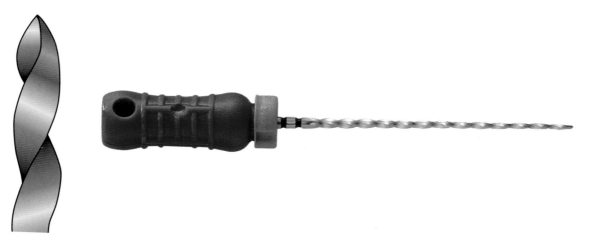

Image courtesy of DENTSPLY Tulsa Dental Specialties, www.tulsadentalspecialties.com

K-FILE

FUNCTION: To remove pulp from canals; smooth and contour canal walls

FEATURES: Stainless steel

TIP SIZES: 6, 8, 10, 15, 20, 25, 30, 35, 40, 45, 50, 55, 60, 70, 80, 90–110, 120–140

LENGTHS: 21, 25, and 30/31 mm

Hand or handpiece driven

TRAY SET-UP: Root canal

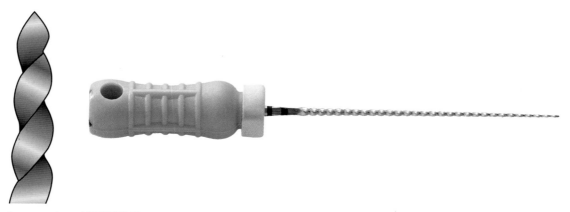

Image courtesy of DENTSPLY Tulsa Dental Specialties, www.tulsadentalspecialties.com

411

HEDSTROM FILE

FUNCTION: To remove pulp from canals; smooth and contour canal walls

FEATURES: Stainless steel
TIP SIZES: 8, 10, 15, 20, 25, 30, 35, 40, 45, 50, 55, 60, 70, 80, 90–110, 120–140
LENGTHS: 21, 25, and 30/31 mm
Hand or handpiece driven

TRAY SET-UP: Root canal

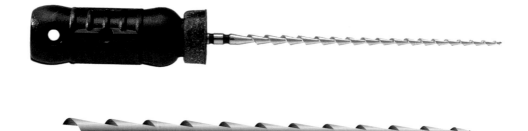

Image courtesy of DENTSPLY Tulsa Dental Specialties, www.tulsadentalspecialties.com

413

NICKEL TITANIUM FILE

FUNCTION: To remove pulp from canals; smooth and contour canal walls

FEATURES: Nickel titanium gives better file flexibility for accessing curved canals

TIP SIZES: 15, 20, 25, 30, 35, 40, 45, 50, 60

LENGTHS: 21, 25, and 30

VARIABLE TIP TAPER: .02, .04, .06, .08, .10

Hand or handpiece driven

TRAY SET-UP: Root canal

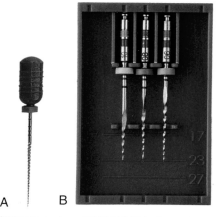

A   B

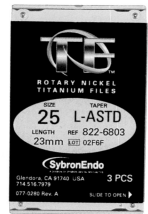

(A) Image courtesy of DENTSPLY Tulsa Dental Specialties, www.tulsadentalspecialties.com and
(B) image courtesy of SybronEndo, www.sybronendo.com

TEST FILE GAUGE

FUNCTION:	To measure and mark length of reamers and files
FEATURES:	Metric rule
	Separate instrument or incorporated into the file organizer
	Some attached to finger ring for easy accessibility
TRAY SET-UP:	Root canal

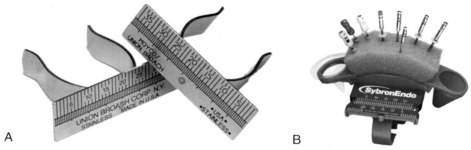

(A) Image courtesy of Miltex, www.miltex.com and (B) image courtesy of SybronEndo, www.sybronendo.com

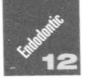

ENDODONTIC STOPS

FUNCTION:	To mark measured length of reamers and files
FEATURES:	1.5-mm-thick silicone disc
	Available in multiple colors
TRAY SET-UP:	Root canal
CLINICAL APPLICATION:	Careful measurement and marking of canal instruments is critical as intracanal instruments must not extend through the apical foramen

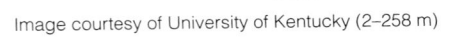

Image courtesy of University of Kentucky (2–258 m)

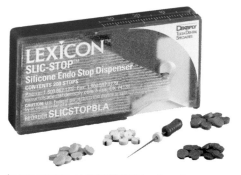

Image courtesy of DENTSPLY Tulsa Dental
Specialties, www.tulsadentalspecialties.com

FILE ORGANIZER

FUNCTION: To hold and organize canal instruments for procedure

FEATURES: Autoclavable plastic or metal

May have built-in metric rule

TRAY SET-UP: Root canal

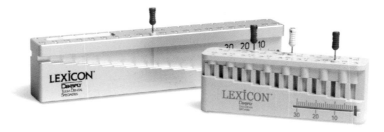

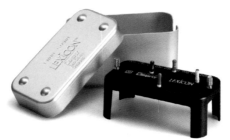

Images courtesy of DENTSPLY Tulsa Dental Specialties, www.tulsadentalspecialties.com

421

PASTE FILLER

FUNCTION: Used in handpiece to place sealer/cement in canal space

TRAY SET-UP: Root canal

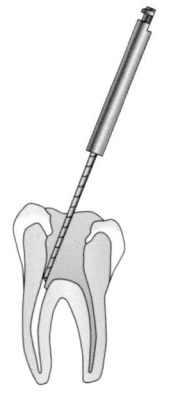

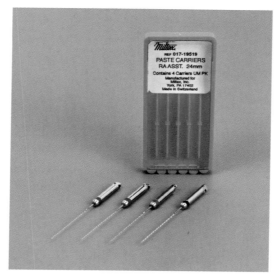

Image courtesy of Miltex, www.miltex.com

ENDO SPREADER

FUNCTION: To laterally condense the filling material (gutta percha) in the canal

TRAY SET-UP: Root canal

CLINICAL APPLICATION: There are three methods of filling the pulp canal:

1. Lateral condensation without heat

2. Warm condensation techniques

3. Core obturator

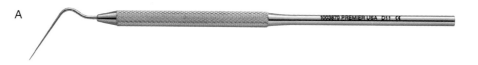

A

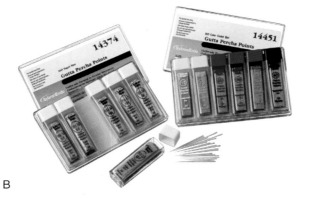

B

(A) Image courtesy of Premier Dental Products, www.premusa.com and (B) image courtesy of SybronEndo, www.sybronendo.com

ENDO PLUGGER

FUNCTION: To laterally and vertically condense the filling material in the canal

Used in the lateral condensation and warm condensation techniques

TRAY SET-UP: Root canal

CLINICAL APPLICATION: There are three methods of filling the pulp canal:

1. Lateral condensation without heat
2. Warm condensation techniques
3. Core obturator

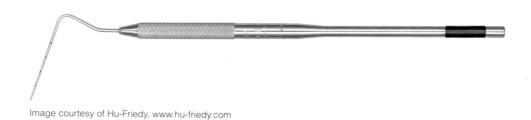

Image courtesy of Hu-Friedy, www.hu-friedy.com

427

Endodontic
12

ENDO-BENDER®

FUNCTION: To bend endodontic instruments to conform to canal curvatures

FEATURES: Safely bends files, pluggers, and spreaders without crimping or breaking instrument
Autoclavable
Numbered gauge

TRAY SET-UP: Root canal

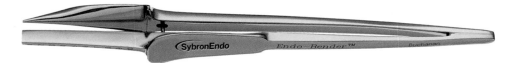

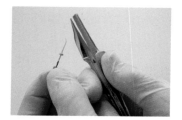

Images courtesy of SybronEndo, www.sybronendo.com

Endodontic
12

HEAT OBTURATION UNIT

FUNCTION: To heat canal-filling material (gutta percha or resin points) for the warm condensation technique.

FEATURES: Unit used to sear and remove excess material, heat master cone and vertically condense ("down pack") material to obtain apical seal and backfill canals

TRAY SET-UP: Root canal

CLINICAL APPLICATION: There are three methods of filling the pulp canal:

1. Lateral condensation without heat

2. Warm condensation techniques

3. Core obturator

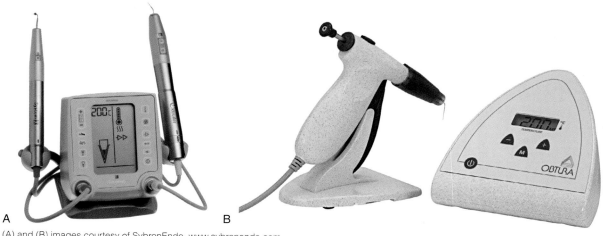

(A) and (B) images courtesy of SybronEndo, www.sybronendo.com

CORE OBTURATOR

FUNCTION: To obtain apical seal and fill canal space

FEATURES: Flexible plastic and titanium carriers coated with plasticized gutta percha
One step filling with heated obturator
BRAND NAMES: Thermafil®, Densfil®, Soft-Core®

TRAY SET-UP: Root canal

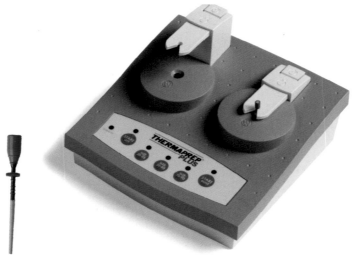

Images courtesy of DENTSPLY Tulsa Dental Specialties,
www.tulsadentalspecialties.com

433

ENDODONTIC PLASTIC INSTRUMENT—GLICK 1

FUNCTION: To place temporary filling materials and to remove excess gutta percha

FEATURES: Elongated plugger on one end and a paddle on the other

TRAY SET-UP: Root canal

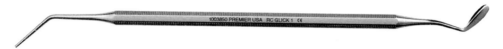

Image courtesy of Premier Dental Products, www.premusa.com

MICRO/RETRO PLACEMENT INSTRUMENT

FUNCTION: To place retrograde filling material

TRAY SET-UP: Apicoectomy

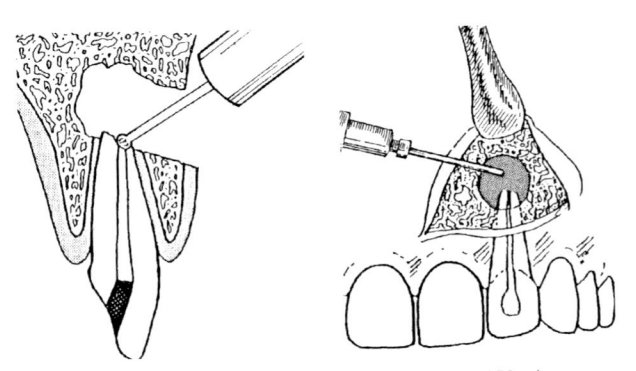

Images courtesy of University of Kentucky (5–259 m, 3–259 m)

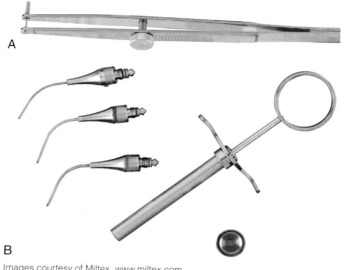

A

B

Images courtesy of Miltex, www.miltex.com

RETRO FILLING INSTRUMENT

FUNCTION: To place and shape retrograde filling material

TRAY SET-UP: Apicoectomy

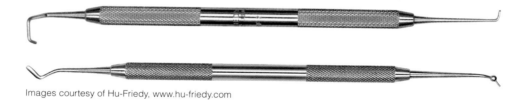

Images courtesy of Hu-Friedy, www.hu-friedy.com

IRRIGATING SYRINGE

FUNCTION: To deliver irrigating solutions to the root canal(s)

Also used to deliver irrigating solutions to a surgical site and for postsurgical at-home irrigation

FEATURES: Plastic syringe in 3 cc 6 cc and 12 cc sizes

Blunt end side-vent needles

TRAY SETUP: Root canal, Apicoectomy

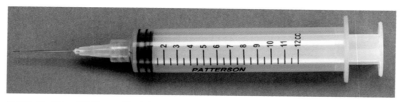

Image courtesy of Patterson Dental, www.pattersondental.com

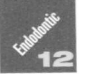

PULP VITALITY TESTER

FUNCTION: Delivers electric stimulus to tooth to determine vitality of pulp

FEATURES: Electric diagnostic unit

Graduated range of electric current settings

Probing tip to place on tooth crown

CLINICAL APPLICATION: Vital, healthy teeth will respond to a low level stimulus without pain. Nonvital teeth generally have minimal or no response to a high-level stimulus. A conductor, such as toothpaste, is applied to the dry tooth surface before placing the probe tip.

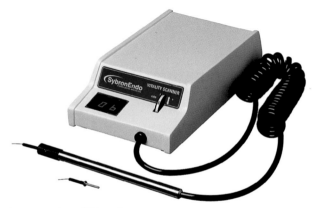

Image courtesy of SybronEndo, www.sybronendo.com

443

APEX LOCATOR

FUNCTION: To locate apex and establish working length of the canal for instrumentation

FEATURES: Electric or battery operated
Audible signal

TRAY SET-UP: Root canal

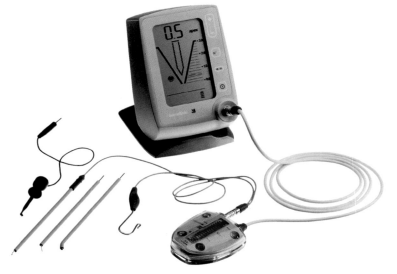

Image courtesy of SybronEndo, www.sybronendo.com

445

ENDODONTIC HANDPIECE

FUNCTION: To hold and rotate rotary endodontic files for enlarging and shaping canal

FEATURES: Torque control motor and/or gear reduction handpiece

CLINICAL APPLICATION: Rotary endodontic files require a handpiece that operates at lower speeds and controls torque, gearing, and direction of rotation. Torque control motors and gear reduction handpieces are utilized to operate endodontic rotary instruments safely and efficiently. Gear reduction contra-angles are available to fit all slow speed handpieces.

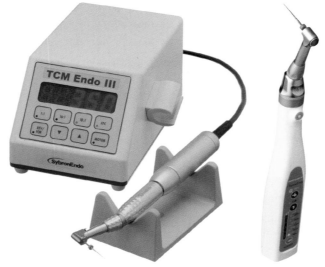

Images courtesy of SybronEndo, www.sybronendo.com

PURPOSE: To provide instrumentation for removing diseased pulp tissue, cleaning and shaping the canal(s), and filling and sealing the canal(s)

1. Dental dam set-up
2. Local anesthesia set-up
3. File gauge
4. Files
5. Stops
6. Burs
7. Intracanal medications
8. Temporary filling material
9. Air/water syringe tip
10. Oral evacuator tip
11. Cotton pliers
12. Endo explorer
13. Endo excavator
14. Endo spreader
15. Endo plugger
16. Endo plastic instrument
17. Irrigating syringe
18. Irrigating solution
19. Paper points
20. Gutta percha points
21. Handpieces (high and low speed)

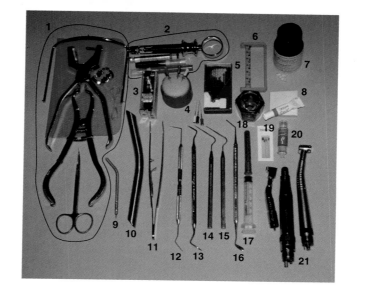

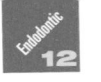

APICOECTOMY SET-UP

PURPOSE: To provide instrumentation for a surgical procedure to remove infection around the apex of the tooth. After making a gingival flap and exposing the apex, a small preparation is made at the end of the root and a restoration placed to seal the canal apically (retrofill).

1. Cotton rolls
2. 2 × 2 gauze
3. Cotton pellets
4. Ultrasonic handpiece and tips
5. Minnesota retractor
6. Adson tissue pliers
7. Local anesthesia syringe
8. Scalpel handles
9. Micro surgical mirror
10. Mouth mirror
11. Explorer
12. Cotton pliers
13. Periodontal probe
14. Endodontic explorer
15. Periosteal elevator
16. Molt curette
17. Gracey curette
18. Cement spatula
19. High speed handpiece
20. Burs
21. Glass slab
22. Retrofill material
23. Micro/retro placement instrument
24. Retro filling instrument
25. Discoid/cleoid
26. Needle holder
27. Iris tissue scissors
28. Surgical aspirating tip

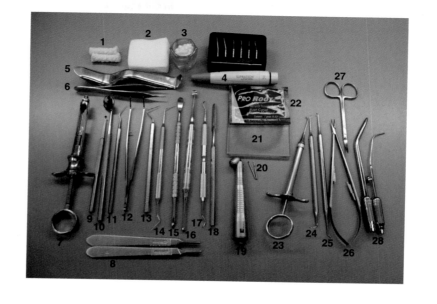

End Chapter 12

PERIODONTAL PROBE

FUNCTION: To measure depth of gingival sulcus, assess gingival bleeding and attachment levels

FEATURES: Cylindrical or flat with blunt end or ball tip

Millimeter markings in variety of increments (3-6-9-12; 1-2-3-5-7-8-9-10; 3-6-8-11; 2-4-6-8-10-12)

Metal probes have notched lines, black or yellow millimeter markings

Plastic probes have green and red millimeter markings

Automated probes also available

TRAY SET-UP: Periodontal exam, prophylaxis, may be part of basic set-up

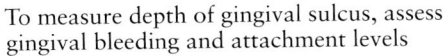

Image courtesy of University of Kentucky (295 m-01)

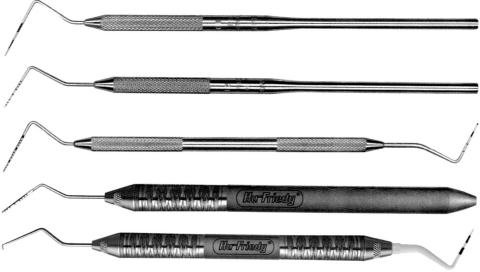

Images courtesy of Hu-Friedy, www.hu-friedy.com

455

FURCATION PERIODONTAL PROBE

FUNCTION: To measure the extent of furcation involvement (loss of bone) on a multirooted tooth

FEATURES: Curved working end

Double ended to allow access to all areas

TRAY SET-UP: Periodontal exam

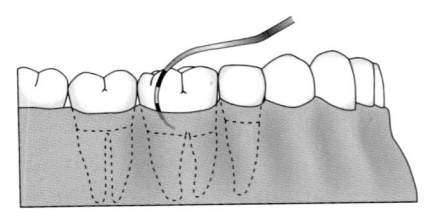

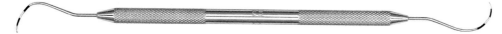

Image courtesy of Hu-Friedy, www.hu-friedy.com

457

SICKLE SCALER—STRAIGHT

FUNCTION: To remove supragingival calculus and cement

FEATURES: Triangular toe ends in a sharp point/tip

Two straight cutting edges on the blade

Usually double ended

Also known as a Jacquette scaler

TRAY SET-UP: Prophylaxis, crown cementation and removal, and orthodontic band cementation and removal

CLINICAL APPLICATION: Scalers are also categorized as (1) anterior or (2) universal. The difference between the two is in the design of the shank. Anterior scalers have a straight shank which limits the adaptability of the instruments. Universal scalers have a curved shank and are double ended to allow access to all areas of the mouth.

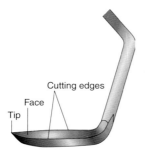

Cutting edges

Face

Tip

Image courtesy of Hu-Friedy, www.hu-friedy.com

459

Hygiene & Periodontal

13

SICKLE SCALER—CURVED

FUNCTION: To remove supragingival calculus and cement

FEATURES: Triangular toe ends in a sharp point

Two curved cutting edges on the blade

Usually double ended

H6/H7, 204S, and U15 are common designs

TRAY SET-UP: Prophylaxis, crown cementation and removal, and orthodontic band cementation and removal

CLINICAL APPLICATION: Scalers are also categorized as (1) anterior or (2) universal. The difference between the two is in the design of the shank. Anterior scalers have a straight shank which limits the adaptability of the instruments. Universal scalers have a curved shank and are double ended to allow access to all areas of the mouth.

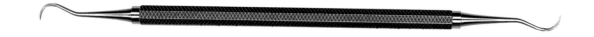

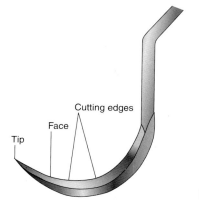

Tip

Face

Cutting edges

Image courtesy of Hu-Friedy, www.hu-friedy.com

HOE SCALER

FUNCTION: To remove heavy, tenacious calculus as an alternative to the ultrasonic scaler

Used on anterior sextants or adjacent to edentulous areas; vertical pull stroke

FEATURES: Single, straight cutting edge

Four designs for the four tooth surfaces—mesial, distal, facial, and lingual

TRAY SET-UP: Prophylaxis

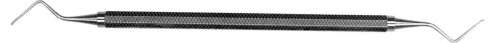

Image courtesy of Hu-Friedy, www.hu-friedy.com

PERIODONTAL FILE

FUNCTION: To crush and remove heavy calculus deposits as an alternative to the ultrasonic scaler; pull stroke

Also used to smooth CEJ and rough or overhanging amalgams

FEATURES: Series of cutting edges on a single base

Hirschfield and Orban designs

TRAY SET-UP: Prophylaxis

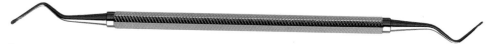

Image courtesy of Hu-Friedy, www.hu-friedy.com

465

IMPLANT SCALER

FUNCTION: Used to remove supragingival calculus without damaging titanium implants

FEATURES: Resin tips that do not scratch titanium

TRAY SET-UP: Prophylaxis

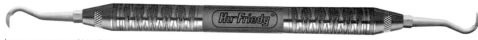

Image courtesy of Hu-Friedy, www.hu-friedy.com

UNIVERSAL CURETTES

FUNCTION: To remove supragingival and subgingival calculus; periodontal debridement

FEATURES: Two cutting edges and a rounded toe

Each instrument can be used on both mesial and distal surfaces in all areas of the mouth

Usually double ended

COMMON DESIGNS: Barnhart, Columbia, Langer, McCall's, Goldman-Fox

TRAY SET-UP: Periodontal debridement (periodontal scaling and root planing), periodontal surgery

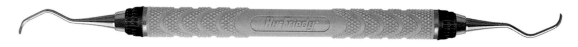

Image courtesy of Hu-Friedy, www.hu-friedy.com

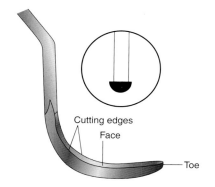

Cutting edges

Face

Toe

469

GRACEY CURETTES (AREA SPECIFIC)

FUNCTION: To remove supragingival and subgingival calculus; periodontal debridement

Designed to permit greater accessibility and adaptability in periodontal treatment

FEATURES: Blade angulation designed for specific surfaces of the tooth and specific areas of the mouth

Angulation of blade allows use of only one cutting edge

Optional rigid shank for removal of heavier calculus

Double ended—1/2, 3/4, 5/6, 7/8, 9/10, 11/12, 13/14, 15/16, 17/18

Variations to standard Gracey curette:

1. 3 mm longer shank for pocket depths of 5 mm or more (After Five™, +3™ Deep Pocket)

2. 3 mm longer shank and 50% shorter blade for greater access in narrow pockets and furcation areas in pocket depths of 5 mm or more (Mini Five™, +3™ Access)

TRAY SET-UP: Periodontal debridement (periodontal scaling and root planing), periodontal surgery

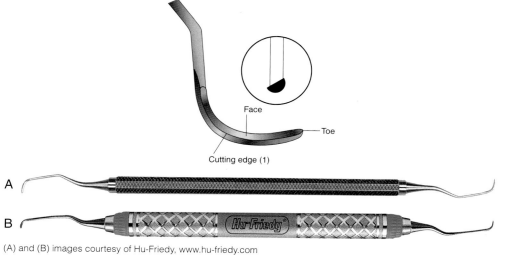

Face

Toe

Cutting edge (1)

A

B

(A) and (B) images courtesy of Hu-Friedy, www.hu-friedy.com

471

PROPHY-JET®

FUNCTION:	To remove dental plaque, soft debris, and stain
FEATURES:	Air polishing system utilizing air pressure to propel water and sodium bicarbonate mixture against tooth surfaces
	Alternative to traditional rubber cup polishing
TRAY SET-UP:	Prophylaxis

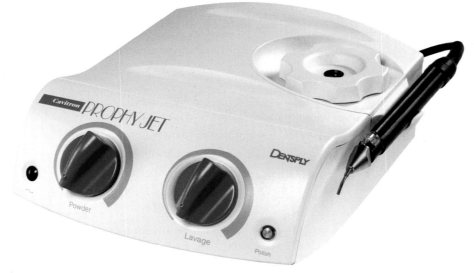

Image courtesy of Dentsply Professional, www.prevent.dentsply.com .

ULTRASONIC SCALER

FUNCTION: To remove supra- and subgingival bacterial plaque and calculus with high frequency sound wave vibrations

FEATURES: Power-driven scaler

Magnetostrictive and piezoelectric types

Handpiece design with tip inserts

Water is supplied to instrument tip to cool tooth and irrigate area

On some models, antimicrobial solutions can also be delivered through the tip inserts to the treatment area

TRAY SET-UP: Prophylaxis, periodontal debridement

CLINICAL APPLICATION: Contraindicated in patients with a communicable disease, immunocompromised individuals and young children. Patient should wear safety glasses and a fluid resistant drape during the procedure.

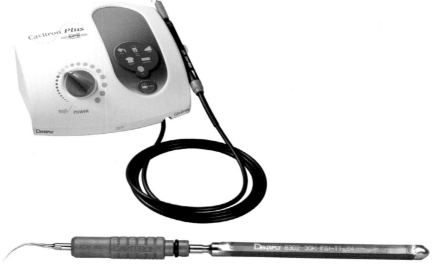

Images courtesy of Dentsply Professional, www.prevent.dentsply.com

475

PERIODONTAL KNIFE

FUNCTION: For initial incision to remove or recontour soft tissue

FEATURES: Common designs: Kirkland, Goldman-Fox

TRAY SET-UP: Gingivectomy and gingivoplasty

Image courtesy of University of Kentucky (4–279 m)

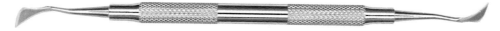

Image courtesy of Hu-Friedy, www.hu-friedy.com

477

INTERDENTAL PERIODONTAL KNIFE

FUNCTION: Spear-pointed blade to remove interproximal tissue

TRAY SET-UP: Gingivectomy and gingivoplasty

Image courtesy of Hu-Friedy, www.hu-friedy.com

479

PERIODONTAL SURGICAL FILE—SUGARMAN

FUNCTION: To recontour and smooth bone in bony pockets

TRAY SET-UP: Osteoplasty

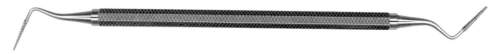

Image courtesy of Hu-Friedy, www.hu-friedy.com

481

PERIODONTAL POCKET MARKER

FUNCTION: To make small holes to mark depth of gingival sulcus and extent of diseased tissue

TRAY SET-UP: Gingivectomy

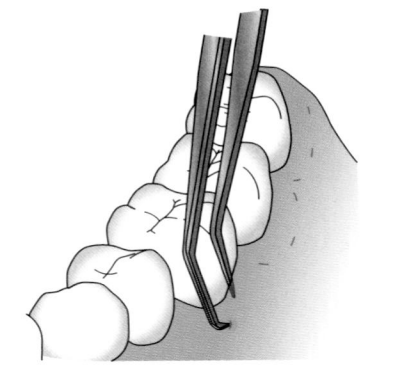

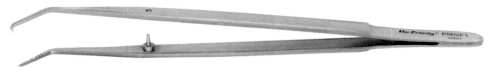

Image courtesy of Hu-Friedy, www.hu-friedy.com

483

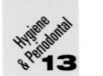

TISSUE NIPPERS

FUNCTION: To remove tissue "tags" and contour interproximal gingiva during soft tissue surgery

TRAY SET-UP: Gingivoplasty

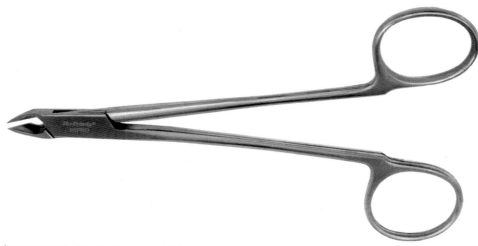

485

Hygiene
& Periodontal
13

PROPHYLAXIS SET-UP

PURPOSE: To provide instrumentation for removing plaque and calculus from tooth surfaces

1. Mouth mirror
2. 5 explorer (combination of #23 and #17)
3. 11/12 explorer
4. Periodontal probe
5. Cotton pliers
6. H6/H7 scaler
7. 204S scaler
8. Prophy handpiece
9. Disposable prophy angle with brush
10. Disposable prophy angle with cup
11. Prophy paste
12. Air/water syringe tip
13. Saliva ejector tip
14. Floss
15. 2 × 2 Gauze

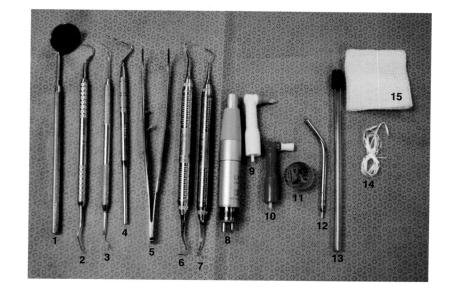

487

SEALANT SET-UP

PURPOSE: To provide instrumentation for preparing tooth surface and placing sealant material on occlusal pits and fissures

1. 2 × 2 Gauze
2. Dri-angles
3. Cotton rolls
4. Disposable prophy angle with brush
5. Prophy handpiece
6. Air/water syringe tip
7. Saliva ejector tip
8. Oral evacuator tip
9. Cotton pliers
10. Mouth mirror
11. Explorer
12. Acid etch, drying agent (optional), sealant material
13. Articulating paper

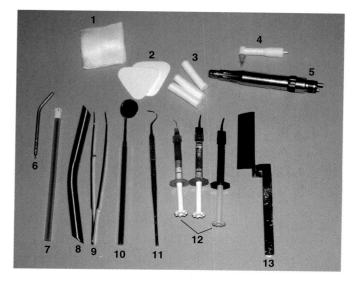

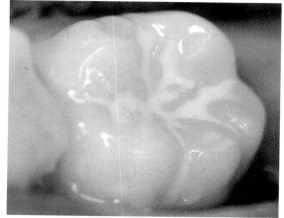

Reprinted with permission from Gladwin MA, Bagby M. Clinical aspects of dental materials: theory, practice, and cases. 3rd ed. Baltimore, MD: Lippincott Williams & Wilkins, 2008.

PERIODONTAL DEBRIDEMENT SET-UP

PURPOSE: To provide instrumentation for removing residual calculus and bacterial toxins from the root surface and gingival wall to promote health and reattachment of the periodontal tissues

1. Local anesthesia set-up
2. Cotton pliers
3. Sharpening stone
4. Mouth mirror
5. 5 explorer (combination of #23 and #17)
6. 11/12 explorer
7. Periodontal probe
8. 204S scaler
9. H6/H7 scaler
10. Gracey curette 1/2
11. Gracey curette 7/8
12. Gracey curette 11/12
13. Gracey curette 13/14
14. Gracey curette 15/16
15. McCalls curette 17/18
16. Air/water syringe tip
17. Oral evacuator tip

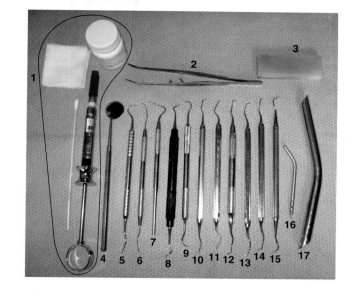

491

GINGIVECTOMY/GINGIVOPLASTY SET-UP

PURPOSE: To provide instrumentation for removing excess/diseased gingiva and for reshaping remaining gingiva to normal contour and marginal outline

1. Local anesthesia set-up
2. 2 × 2 Gauze
3. High-speed handpiece
4. Diamonds/burs
5. Suture
6. Tissue nippers
7. Iris tissue scissors
8. Periodontal dressing
9. Sharpening stone
10. Cotton pliers
11. Mouth mirror
12. 11/12 Explorer
13. Periodontal probe
14. Periodontal pocket marker
15. Periodontal knife
16. Interdental knife
17. H6/H7 scaler
18. 204S scaler
19. Gracey curette 1/2
20. Gracey curette 7/8
21. Gracey curette 11/12
22. Gracey curette 13/14
23. Gracey curette 15/16
24. McCalls curette 17/18
25. Surgical aspirating tip
26. Hemostat/needle holder

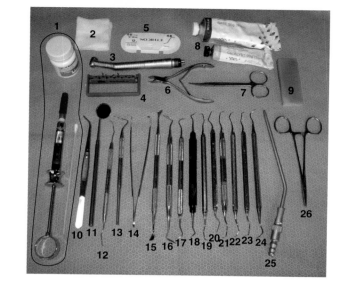

OSTEOPLASTY

OSTEOPLASTY

PURPOSE: To provide instrumentation for removing bony defects caused by periodontal disease and for reshaping remaining bone

1. Local anesthesia set-up
2. 2 × 2 Gauze
3. High-speed handpiece
4. Diamonds/burs
5. Tissue nippers
6. Iris tissue scissors
7. Suture
8. Periodontal dressing
9. Sharpening stone
10. Mouth mirror
11. 11/12 Explorer
12. Cotton pliers
13. Scalpel
14. Periosteal elevator
15. Tissue retractor
16. Periodontal knife
17. Interdental knife
18. H6/H7 scaler
19. 204S scaler
20. Gracey curette 1/2
21. Gracey curette 7/8
22. Gracey curette 11/12
23. Gracey curette 13/14
24. Gracey curette 15/16
25. McCalls curette 17/18
26. Sugarman periodontal file
27. Hirschfield periodontal file
28. Surgical aspirating tip
29. Hemostat/needle holder

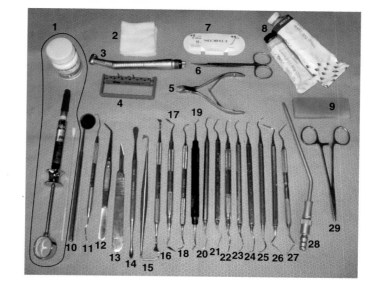

End Chapter 13

Orthodontic
Instruments

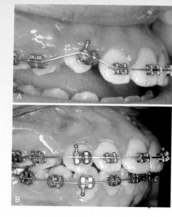

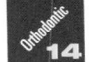

UTILITY PLIERS—WEINGART

FUNCTION: General purpose plier used to place and remove archwires

Also used for placement of bands, brackets, and auxiliaries

FEATURES: Angled, serrated tips

TRAY SET-UP: Archwire adjustment and tie-in, banding and bonding

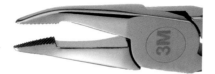

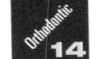

UTILITY PLIERS—HOW

FUNCTION:	To place and remove archwires
	Also used for placement of bands, brackets, and auxiliaries
FEATURES:	Serrated tips
	Angled or straight tip designs
TRAY SET-UP:	Archwire adjustment and tie-in, banding and bonding

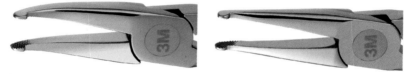

501

Orthodontic
14

WIRE BENDING PLIERS—BIRD BEAK

FUNCTION: To bend and contour orthodontic wires

FEATURES: One round tip, one pyramid-shaped tip
Short- and long-tip designs

TRAY SET-UP: Archwire adjustment and tie-in

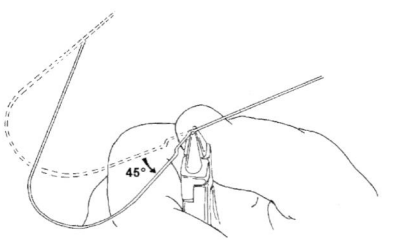

Image courtesy of University of Kentucky
(806 or -08)

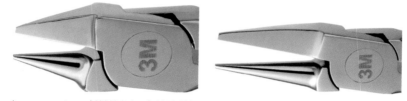

WIRE BENDING PLIERS—OPTICAL

FUNCTION:	To bend and contour orthodontic wires
FEATURES:	Long, round tips
	Adjusts all types of loops
TRAY SET-UP:	Archwire adjustment and tie-in

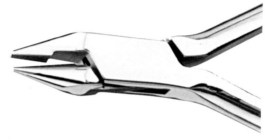

Image courtesy of Dentronix, www.dentronix.com

505

WIRE BENDING PLIERS—ARCH BENDING

FUNCTION: To torque and bend archwire

TRAY SET-UP: Archwire adjustment and tie-in

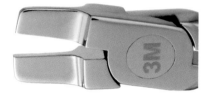

507

Orthodontic
14

WIRE BENDING PLIERS—LOOP FORMING

FUNCTION: To make various loops in archwires

TRAY SET-UP: Archwire adjustment and tie-in

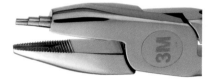

509

WIRE BENDING PLIERS—3-PRONG

FUNCTION: To bend and contour orthodontic wires, especially clasp and appliance adjustment

TRAY SET-UP: Appliance adjustment

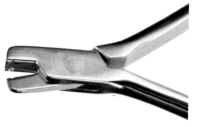

Image courtesy of Dentronix,
www.dentronix.com

511

CONTOURING PLIERS

FUNCTION: To contour bands and temporary crowns in cervical area

FEATURES: "Bird beak" and "ball and socket" designs

TRAY SET-UP: Band seating, crown prep

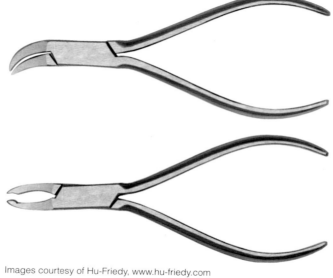

Images courtesy of Hu-Friedy, www.hu-friedy.com

513

WIRE CUTTER—PIN AND LIGATURE CUTTER

FUNCTION: To cut soft wires and ligatures

TRAY SET-UP: Archwire adjustment and tie-in

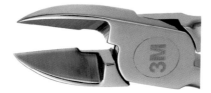

WIRE CUTTER—DISTAL END CUTTER

FUNCTION: To cut archwires

FEATURES: Designed to cut and safely hold the cut end of a tied-in archwire

TRAY SET-UP: Archwire adjustment and tie-in

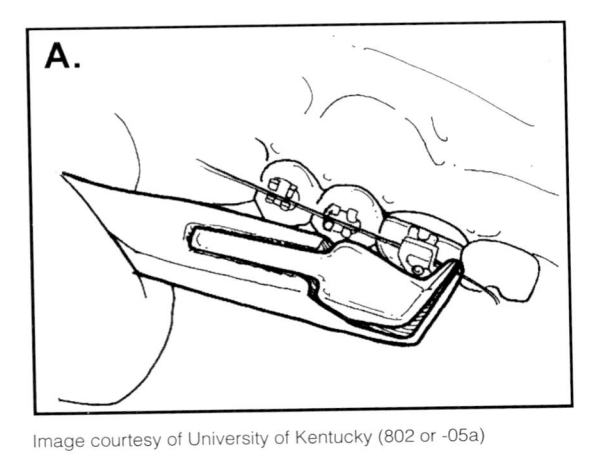

Image courtesy of University of Kentucky (802 or -05a)

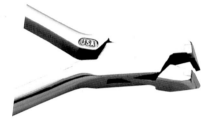

Image courtesy of Dentronix,
www.dentronix.com

517

WIRE CUTTER—HARD WIRE CUTTER

FUNCTION: To cut archwires before placement

TRAY SET-UP: Archwire adjustment and tie-in

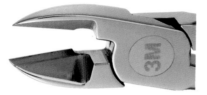

Orthodontic
14

SEPARATING PLIERS

FUNCTION: To place separators

TRAY SET-UP: Preliminary appointment prior to band fitting and seating

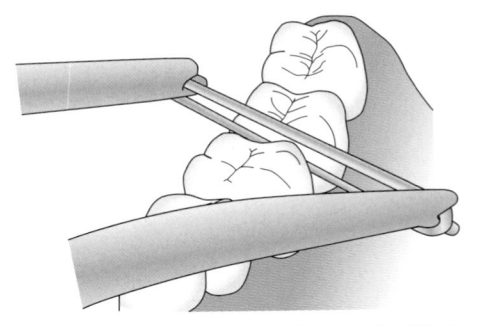

Image modified from university of kentucky (1–269m)

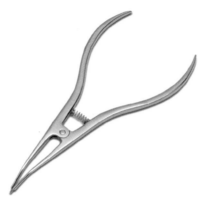

Orthodontic
14

LIGATURE TYING PLIERS

FUNCTION: To tie/twist ligature wires around brackets to secure archwire

FEATURES: Slots in working ends securely hold ligature wires for tying archwire into bracket

TRAY SET-UP: Archwire adjustment and tie-in

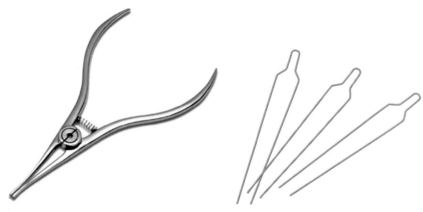

Image courtesy of Hu-Friedy, www.
hu-friedy.com

523

LIGATURE TUCKER/DIRECTOR

FUNCTION: To tuck the cut ends of the ligature wires under the archwire

FEATURES: Notched tips for tucking wires

Flat serrated ends for tucking wires and assisting in placement of elastic ligatures

Curved pointed ends for removing elastic ligatures

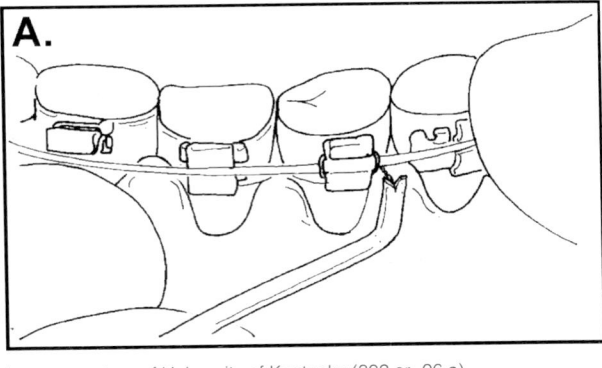

Image courtesy of University of Kentucky (802 or -06 a)

TRAY SET-UP: Archwire adjustment and tie-in

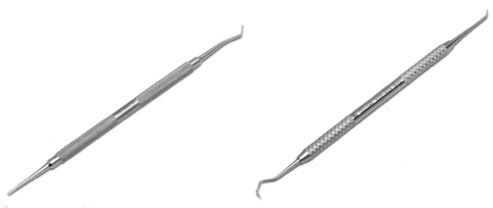

525

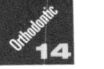

MATHIEU PLIERS

FUNCTION: To place elastic auxiliaries

FEATURES: Quick-release locking mechanism on handles

TRAY SET-UP: Archwire adjustment and tie-in

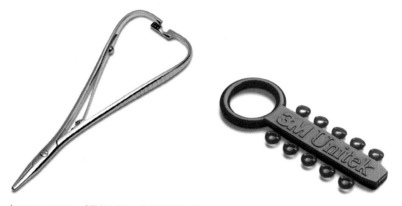

BAND PUSHERS

FUNCTION: To place orthodontic bands with hand pressure

TRAY SET-UP: Band fitting and seating

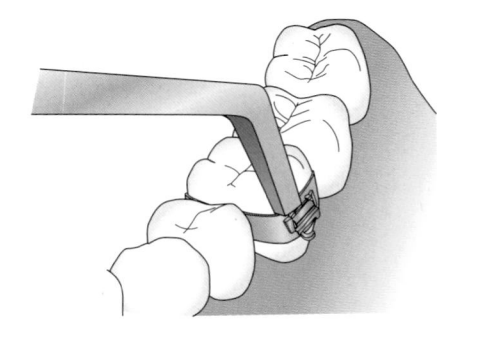

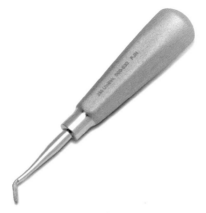

Image courtesy of 3M Unitek—
© 2010 3M. All rights reserved.
www.3MUnitek.com

BAND SEATERS ("BITE STICK")

FUNCTION: To place orthodontic bands with biting pressure

TRAY SET-UP: Band fitting and seating

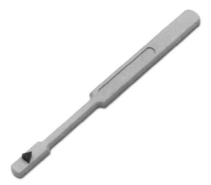

BAND FILE

FUNCTION: To shape bands, burnish and remove burs, and mark archwires

TRAY SET-UP: Band fitting and seating

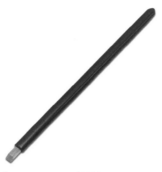

BRACKET PLACEMENT MARKER—BOONE POSITIONING GAUGE

FUNCTION: To determine correct placement of brackets

TRAY SET-UP: Bracket placement and bonding

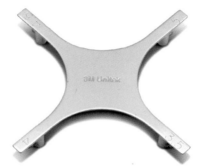

BONDING TWEEZERS

FUNCTION: To hold bracket for accurate placement during bonding procedure

TRAY SET-UP: Bracket placement and bonding

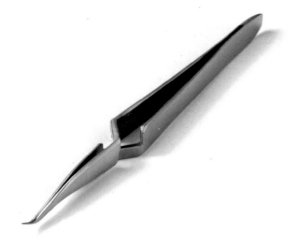

BAND REMOVING PLIERS

FUNCTION: To remove orthodontic bands

TRAY SET-UP: Debanding/debonding

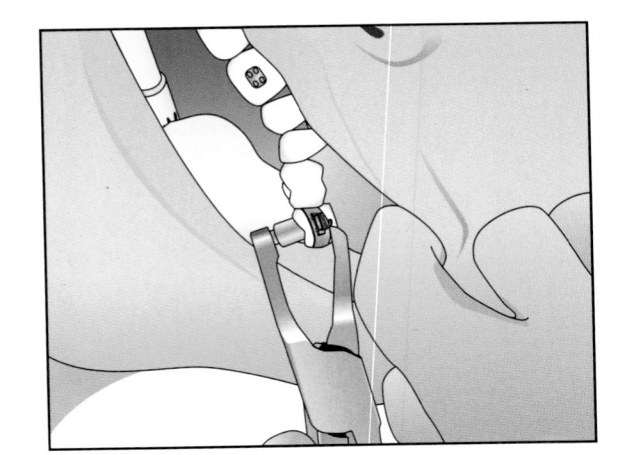

Image modified from University of Kentucky (804 or -05)

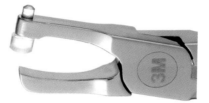

Image courtesy of 3M Unitek—© 2010 3M.
All rights reserved. www.3MUnitek.com

539

Orthodontic
14

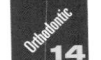

DEBONDING PLIERS/INSTRUMENT

FUNCTION: To remove orthodontic brackets

TRAY SET-UP: Bracket removal/debonding

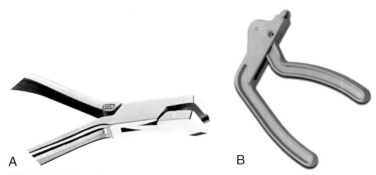

A   B

BOND REMOVER PLIERS

FUNCTION: To remove bonding and composite materials

TRAY SET-UP: Bracket removal/debonding

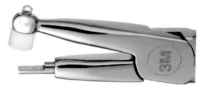

Orthodontic
14

PLACEMENT OF ELASTIC SEPARATORS SET-UP

PURPOSE: To provide instrumentation for placement of separators at mesial and distal contacts of first permanent molars to create space for seating orthodontic band

1. Mouth mirror
2. Explorer
3. Cotton pliers
4. Separating pliers
5. Elastic separators
6. Floss
7. Air/water syringe tip
8. Saliva ejector tip

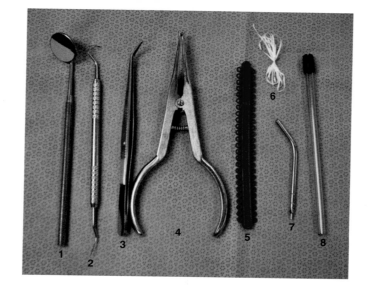

BAND SEATING AND BRACKET BONDING SET-UP

PURPOSE: To provide instrumentation to fit, position, cement/bond bands and brackets, and tie-in initial archwire

1. Brackets and bands on organizer
2. Cement guard
3. Boone positioning gauge
4. Archwire
5. Elastic ligatures
6. Floss
7. Mouth mirror
8. Explorer
9. Cotton pliers
10. Band pusher
11. Band seater
12. Band removing pliers
13. Weingart utility pliers
14. Wire bending pliers
15. Wire cutter
16. Mathieu pliers
17. Distal end cutter
18. Air/water syringe tip
19. Saliva ejector tip

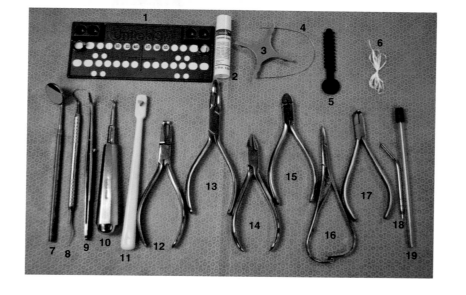

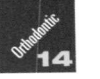
ARCHWIRE ADJUSTMENT AND TIE-IN SET-UP

PURPOSE: To provide instrumentation for archwire adjustment or replacement at periodic intervals

1. Archwire
2. Elastic ligatures
3. Floss
4. Mouth mirror
5. Explorer
6. Cotton pliers
7. Scaler
8. Weingart utility pliers
9. Wire bending pliers
10. Wire cutter
11. Mathieu pliers
12. Distal end cutter
13. Air/water syringe tip
14. Saliva ejector tip

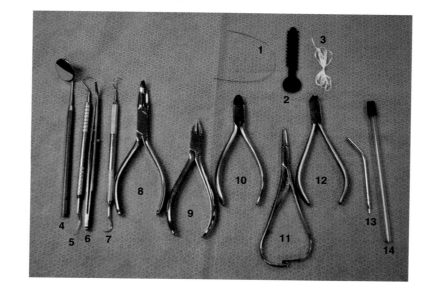

549

DEBANDING/DEBONDING SET-UP

PURPOSE: To provide instrumentation for removing bands and brackets at completion of treatment

1. Finishing burs, polishing points, and discs
2. Contra-angle handpiece attachment
3. Prophy handpiece
4. Prophy paste
5. Disposable prophy angle with cup
6. Floss
7. Mouth mirror
8. Explorer
9. Cotton pliers
10. Scaler
11. Weingart utility pliers
12. Band removing pliers
13. Debracketing instrument
14. Air/water syringe tip
15. Saliva ejector tip
16. Oral evacuator tip

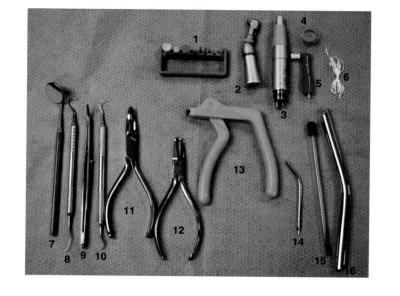

End Chapter 14

Chapter 15

Radiographic Instruments and Equipment

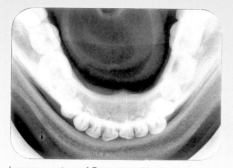

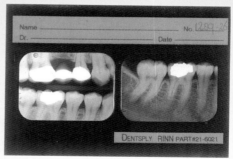

Images courtesy of Carestream Health, Inc., www.kodakdental.com

INTRAORAL FILM

FUNCTION: To record images of teeth and oral structures

FEATURES: Plastic (poly) or paper packets

Available with clear barrier packets

Color-coded single and double film packets

Sizes: 0, 1, 2, 3, 4

Film speed D and F

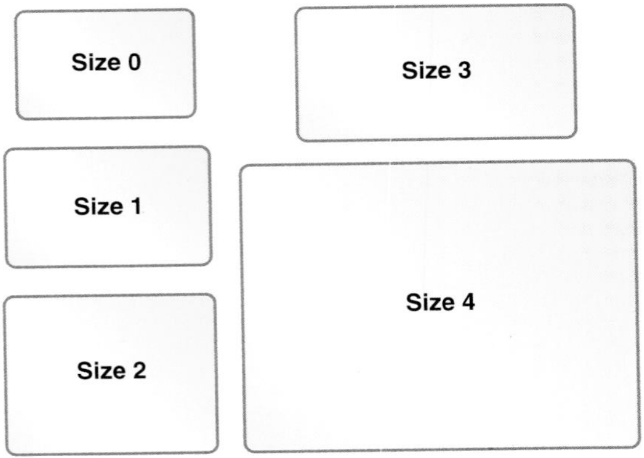

Size 0

Size 1

Size 2

Size 3

Size 4

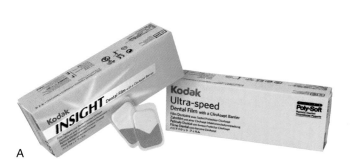

A

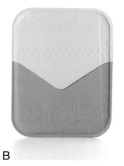

B

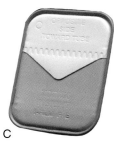

C

(A) Kodak film packages with ClinAsept barrier film packets, (B) Insight film packet, and (C) Suresoft film packet courtesy of Carestream Health, Inc., www.kodakdental.com

INTRAORAL DIGITAL SENSORS

FUNCTION: To record images of teeth and oral structures using digital technology

FEATURES: **1.** Phosphor storage plates

Sizes: 0, 1, 2, 3, 4

Similar in size and shape to conventional intraoral film

Image is stored on sensor and then scanned to computer

2. CCD sensor

Sizes 1 and 2

Wired sensor

Image is immediately sent to computer

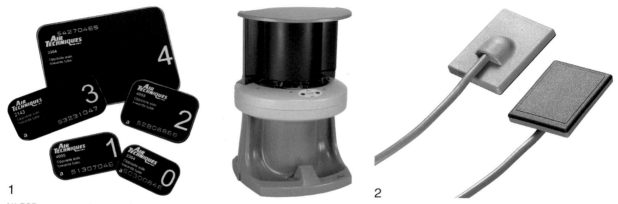

1

2

(1) PSP sensors and scanner for PSP sensors and (2) CCD sensors courtesy of Air Techniques, Inc., www.airtechniques.com

FILM HOLDERS

FUNCTION: To stabilize film in patient's mouth during exposure

COMMON TYPES:
1. Snap-A-Ray (formerly EEZEE Grip)
2. Rinn XCP
3. Stabe
4. Bitewing tabs—pressure sensitive or loop style

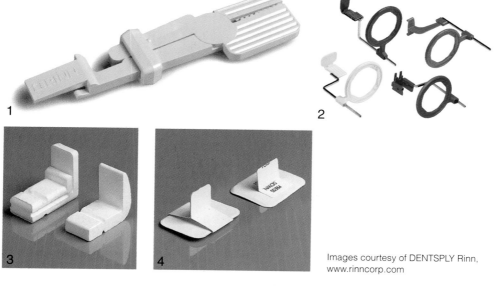

1

2

3

4

Images courtesy of DENTSPLY Rinn,
www.rinncorp.com

INTRAORAL X-RAY SYSTEM

FUNCTION: To provide x-rays for film and digital sensor exposure

FEATURES: Adjustable exposure values—preprogrammed and manual
Mobile and wall mounted

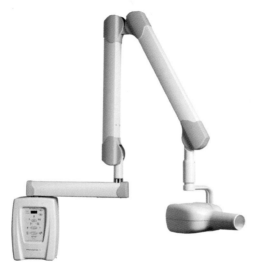

Image courtesy of Air Techniques, Inc.,
www.airtechniques.com

PANORAMIC AND CEPHALOMETRIC IMAGING SYSTEM

FUNCTION: To provide x-rays for film and digital sensor exposure
To position patient and film/digital sensor for exposure
Digital and film based

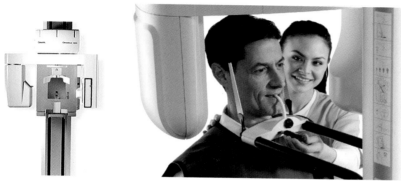

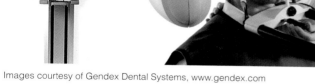

Images courtesy of Gendex Dental Systems, www.gendex.com

CONE BEAM 3D IMAGING

FUNCTION: To capture anatomically correct 3D images of oral and facial structures

FEATURES: Digital extraoral imaging system

Provides information not visible in traditional two-dimensional images

Used in implant treatment planning, temporomandibular joint analysis, oral and maxillofacial surgery, orthodontic treatment planning, and other dental procedures

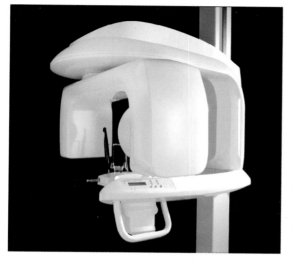

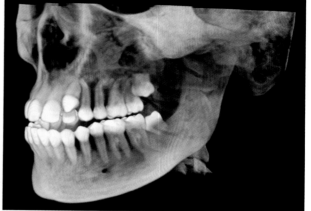

Images courtesy of Carestream Health, Inc., www.kodakdental.com

AUTOMATIC PROCESSOR

FUNCTION:	Automates all film processing steps
	Transports unwrapped dental film through the developer, fixer, water, and drying chamber and into film recovery slots
FEATURES:	Roller and rollerless transport systems
	Daylight loader option
	Some process only intraoral film sizes; other models process both intraoral and extraoral films
CLINICAL APPLICATION:	Regular preventive maintenance and a closely followed cleaning and replenishment schedule are necessary to ensure optimum performance and prevent malfunctioning of an automatic processor.

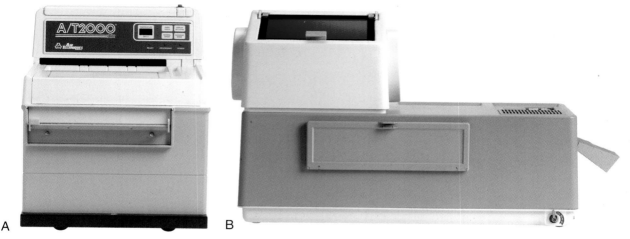

(A) A/T 2000 and (B) Peri-Pro® III with daylight loader courtesy of Air Techniques.

End Chapter 15

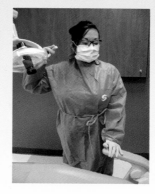

PERSONAL PROTECTIVE EQUIPMENT (PPE)—CLINIC JACKET/LAB COAT AND GLOVES

FUNCTION: To protect health care workers' skin from contact with pathogens and chemicals during treatment procedures, treatment room decontamination, and instrument processing

GLOVE FEATURES:

1. Exam gloves
Latex, nitrile, or vinyl
Powdered or powder free
Sizes: XS, S, M, L, XL

2. Surgical gloves
Sterile latex, nitrile, or chloroprene
Right/left hand specific
Powdered or powder free
Sizes: 5 1/2, 6, 6 1/2, 7, 7 1/2, 8, 8 1/2, 9

3. Utility gloves
Heavyweight nitrile for sterilization
and disinfection procedures
Sizes: S, M, L, XL

4. Overgloves
Disposable clear plastic
Sizes: S, M, L

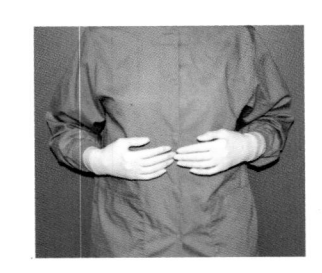

JACKET FEATURES: Moisture resistant disposable or cloth

Long, cuffed sleeves

Crew neck with snap or button closure

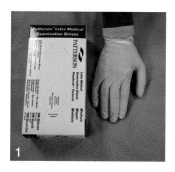

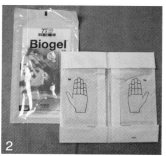

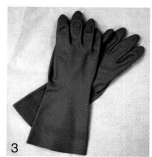

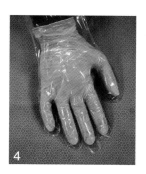

PERSONAL PROTECTIVE EQUIPMENT (PPE)—MASKS AND PROTECTIVE GLASSES

FUNCTION:	To protect health care workers' mucous membranes from contact with airborne pathogens, debris and chemicals during treatment procedures, treatment room decontamination, and instrument processing
MASK FEATURES:	Covers nose and mouth
	Earloop, molded cup, and surgical tie-on styles
	Fluid resistant outer layer
	Varying filtration rates
GLASSES FEATURES:	Impact resistant
	Wrap around or with side shields for full coverage
	Variety of sizes and styles available

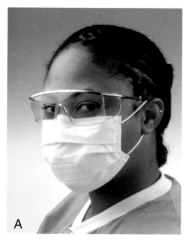 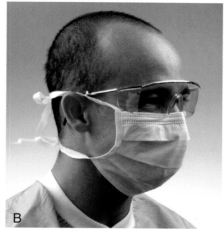 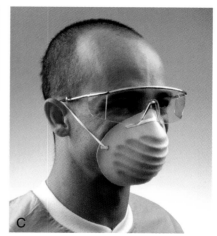

(A) Earloop mask, (B) tie-on mask, and (C) molded cup with elastic band courtesy of Crosstex, www.crosstex.com

INSTRUMENT CASSETTES

FUNCTION: To organize instruments for use at chairside

To hold instruments during cleaning and sterilization procedures

FEATURES: Constructed of metal or heat resistant resin

Many sizes and designs to accommodate different number and shapes of instruments

CLINICAL APPLICATION: Cassettes are an efficient way to organize instruments in functional sets for treatment procedures, decontamination and sterilization, and storage. Cassettes hold the instruments during use at chairside. Following the procedure, instruments remain in the closed cassette during cleaning and packaging for sterilization.

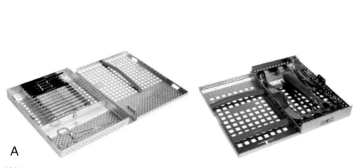
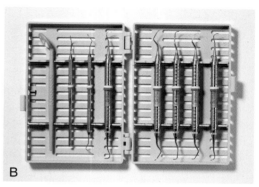

(A) Image courtesy of American Eagle Instruments, Inc., www.am-eagle.com, and (B) image courtesy of Dux Dental, www.duxdental.com

Infection
Control
16

INSTRUMENT WRAP AND PACKAGING

FUNCTION: To package instrument cassettes and single or grouped instruments for sterilization

Maintains sterility of instruments during storage and until time of use

FEATURES: Nonwoven, moisture resistant CSR wrap for use with steam, chemical vapor, and ethylene oxide (EO) gas (some can also be used with dry heat)

Steam permeable paper and paper/plastic pouches available in various sizes for use with steam, chemical vapor, or EO gas

Nylon tubing available for use with dry heat, chemical vapor, and steam

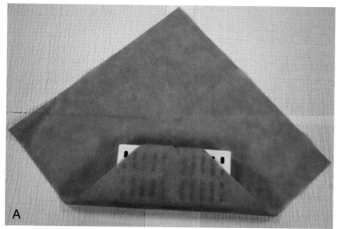

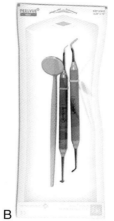

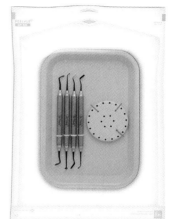

(A) and (B) images courtesy of Dux Dental, www.duxdental.com

ULTRASONIC CLEANER

FUNCTION: To remove debris from instruments in preparation for sterilization

Also used to remove debris from dentures and other dental appliances before disinfection

FEATURES: Interior removable basket to hold instruments during debris removal cycle and during rinsing

Timed cycle

One gallon and 3 gallon size

CLINICAL APPLICATION: Ultrasonic cleaners are not sterilizers. Utility gloves should be worn when placing instruments in the ultrasonic and when rinsing and drying them because the "cleaned" instruments are still contaminated. Always place the lid on the ultrasonic during the cleaning cycle to reduce airborne contaminants and splash. The ultrasonic solution should be changed at least once a day.

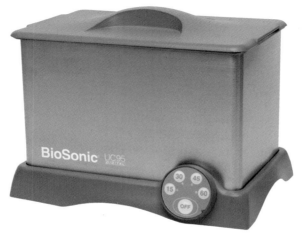

Image courtesy of Coltene Whaledent, www.coltene.com

STERILIZERS

FUNCTION: To destroy all microbes on dental instruments

DENTAL STERILIZERS:
1. Steam autoclave
2. Unsaturated chemical vapor sterilizer
3. Dry heat sterilizer—oven type or rapid heat transfer
4. Ethylene Oxide (EO) gas sterilization is primarily used in hospitals and industry, very minimal use in dentistry. (not pictured)

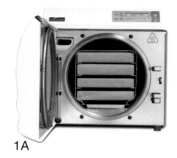

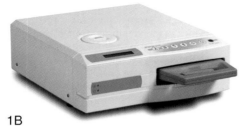

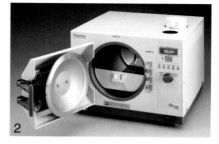

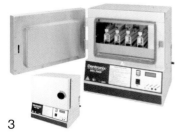

(1a) UltraClave® courtesy of Midmark Corporation, www.midmark.com; (1b) STATIM 2000 courtesy of SciCan, www.scican.ca; (2) Harvey Chemiclave courtesy of Thermo Scientific, www.thermo.com; and (3) DDS 7000 courtesy of Dentronix, www.dentronix.com

BIOLOGICAL INDICATORS (BIs)

FUNCTION: Sterilization indicator

Monitors sterilization process by assessing destruction of highly resistant microbes

FEATURES: Spore strips or ampules of nonpathogenic bacterial spores (geobacillus stearothermophilus and/or bacillus atrophaeus spores)

Also known as spore tests

CLINICAL APPLICATION: Weekly biological monitoring is recommended by the Centers for Disease Control (CDC) and the Organization for Safety, Asepsis and Prevention (OSAP). A biological monitor (BI) is placed inside an instrument package and sterilized with other instrument packages under normal circumstances. After the sterilization cycle the processed BI and a control BI (one not exposed to sterilization process) are sent to an independent monitoring service or the BIs can be incubated in-office with a dry block incubator. A negative result indicates that sterilization occurred, all spores destroyed. A positive result indicates a sterilization failure, spores survived.

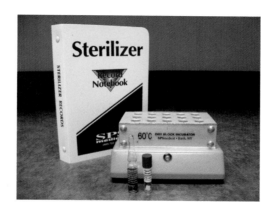

Infection
Control
16

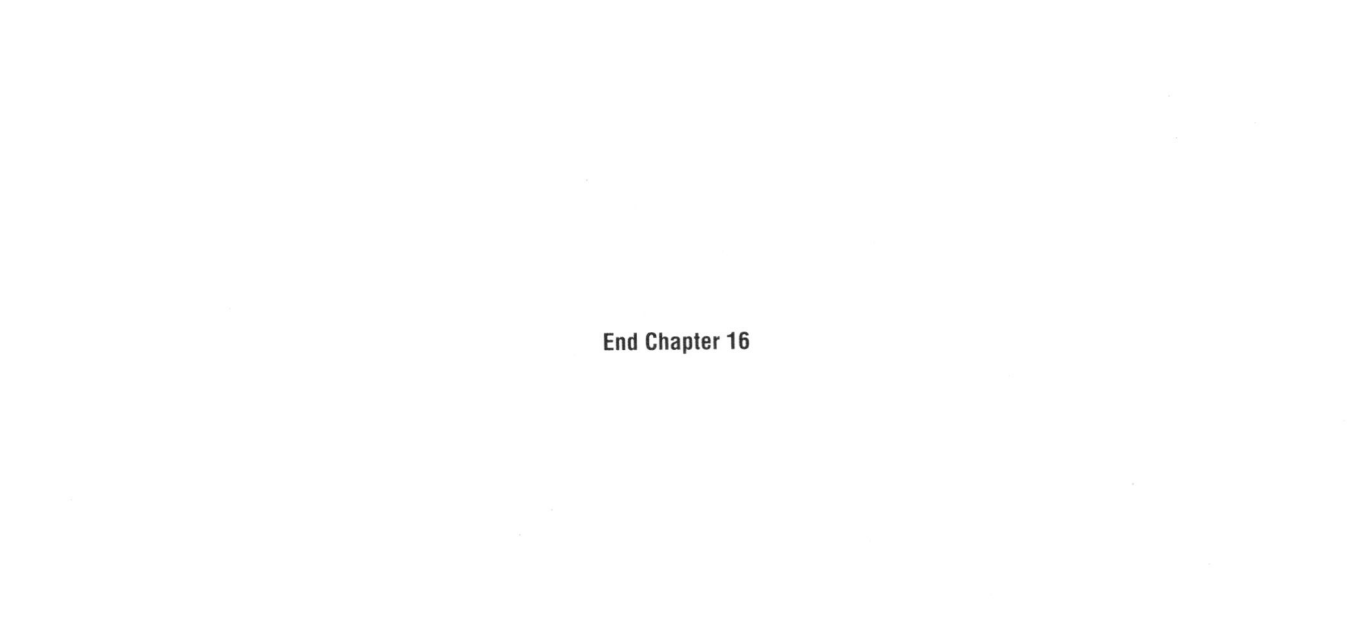

End Chapter 16

Index

Note: Page locators followed by f indicates figures.

585